I0222619

DIVORCING FITNESS

FOR A
BETTER RELATIONSHIP
WITH HEALTH

TODD HELLMER

Copyright © 2020 by Todd Hellmer

All rights reserved. No part of this publication may be reproduced, distributed, or transmitted in any form or by any means, including photocopying, recording, or other electronic or mechanical methods, without the prior written permission of the publisher, except in the case of brief quotations embodied in critical reviews and certain other noncommercial uses permitted by copyright law. For permission requests, write to the publisher, addressed "Attention: Permissions Coordinator," at info@divorcingfitness.com

Published by 4S1 Health.
Contact 4S1 Health at info@divorcingfitness.com

ISBN: 978-1-7330167-0-4 (print)
ISBN: 978-1-7330167-1-1(ebook)

Ordering Information:
Special discounts are available on quantity purchases by corporations, associations, and others. For details, contact info@divorcingfitness.com

Divorcing Fitness ™ Todd Hellmer
Cover design by Michael Korber
Drawings on rear cover and introducing Part 2 © Michael Korber

To share a story about fitness, contact the author at todd@divorcingfitness.com

The author of this book is not a licensed or certified musculoskeletal or medical practitioner. This book was written as a researcher and based on personal observation. This entire book is informational and should not be considered medical advice or instruction. No decision or indecision to act or not act should be taken solely based on this book. Any action taken without consultation of a licensed professional or doctor is done so with the assumption of risk.

CONTENTS

Introduction 1

Part 1: How Bad Fitness Relationships Take Shape.................. 5
Chapter 1: There's No You in Fitness....................................... 7
Chapter 2: How Marketing and Culture Obscure Health...................... 17
Chapter 3: Tuning in to Your Body and Mind.................................. 27

Part 2: Your Fitness Past—Where Is It Leading You?.............. 39
Chapter 4: Are You Ignoring Your Body?................................. 41
Chapter 5: Complete Program or "Sexy" Muscle Focus?........................ 55
Chapter 6: Are Your Cardio Habits as Healthy as You Think?.............. 65
Chapter 7: How Did Others Influence Your Motivation? 73
Chapter 8: Performance or Health—What Matters More? 81
Chapter 9: Did Fitness Get Physically or Emotionally Painful?............. 89
Chapter 10: Have Ads Blocked Long-Term Health Goals? 97

Summary: Are You on a Healthy Fitness Path? 101

Part 3: Things to Learn and Accept Before Moving On........ 105
Chapter 11: Ads Did Not Get Us Emotional About Health 107
Chapter 12: Fitness Biases Are Real and Limit Health 115
Chapter 13: Why Habits Are a Bigger Deal than We Think 121

Part 4: Pivot Toward Your Health-First Fitness Future 131
Chapter 14: Setting Your Goals, Your Club, Your Clock...................... 133
Chapter 15: Weight Loss Habits that Start with You 143
Chapter 16: Becoming Body Aware, Focusing on Weak Links............. 161
Chapter 17: Building Your Complete Program................................. 181

Part 5: Exercises for Today, Tomorrow,
and the Rest of Your Life.. 195

Introduction

Do **you know** the joint health of Americans has been so bad for so long that the government launched a US Joint and Bone Initiative (USJBI) in 2002? Here are the first words on the USJBI website home page:

"Movement, for nearly one in two Americans over the age of 18, and many children, is restricted by a musculoskeletal disorder—arthritis, back pain, fracture, osteoporosis, sports trauma, and other ailments which affect function and mobility."

That's half of adults and many children!

The trend is not favorable. The costs of musculoskeletal disorders were approximately $400 billion between 1996 and 1998. That number more than doubled to over $800 billion between 2012 and 2014.[1] For comparison, consider that the United States military spent $571 billion in 2014.[2]

Do you know that many of our common exercise habits won't correct these minor or major disorders and that our most common exercise habits can cause or exacerbate them? Yep. Exercise can and should prevent musculoskeletal disorders. Instead, exercise as many do it helps fuel a rising social health burden.

Finally, do you know that many of us are so emotional about our looks, performance, and social fitness goals that joint health is either not considered, ignored, or deprioritized?

Learning and accepting these facts radically improved my health. It can change yours.

I didn't want to divorce fitness. I had to. I slowly developed health issues from my feet to my neck. Like many others, pursing looks, social and performance-related goals in fitness was a major source of these joint health problems. I was a fitness enthusiast for 30 years and a fitness group exercise instructor for 15 of those 30, teaching multiple types of classes as a hobby in my twenties and thirties at over 10 gyms in Chicago. Then, in my forties, I divorced fitness and took a needed step back. I made the long-term health of my body essential to living a healthy life with my wife, Lorraine, my number one priority.

I walked away from my favorite exercises. I became passionate about researching fitness for joint health to find a program that would work for my body. I had to learn a lot of things that the fitness culture doesn't teach us.

I'll share what I learned from my joint research and personal history with fitness to show how fitness can cause or exacerbate chronic health issues, even doing simple things like cardio.

I'll also share how to navigate the musculoskeletal health care system as a proactive driver instead of a reactive passenger. Too many of us don't proactively use this system to become aware of our bodies and to find key exercises that can transform our health.

It doesn't matter if you are a super fitness enthusiast, a novice, or if you don't exercise at all. It doesn't matter if you are injured or not. You likely can get a little or a lot more out of fitness if you learn how to exercise for your body.

It may seem odd to question that fitness can be unhealthy. It can be, however, when we let fitness marketing and culture steer our motivation away from health and when we believe that exercise plays a bigger role in weight loss than it does or should. It also can be unhealthy when we knowingly or unwittingly ignore generally available information on joint health and how to prevent joint issues, just like we ignored generally available information on the dangers of smoking after the US Surgeon General's warning in 1964 about the dangers of smoking.[3]

I believe that we care about long-term joint health today and the impact of sports and fitness on it, similarly to how we cared about the impact of long-term health from cigarette smoking in the mid-1960s. This was a time when many people, particularly young people, had positive emotional associations with smoking and were influenced by marketing and culture. The same is true today with fitness.

My eclectic background in sales strategy, market analysis (University of Chicago MBA), product marketing, neuro market research technology (which drove lots of reading on habits and behavioral science), love of science (electrical engineering undergrad), fascination with human motivation, fitness experience, and joint research to reclaim my body is a unique mix to see fitness through a new lens. One where you can look at your past experiences with fitness marketing and culture to assess the degree to which your current motivation for and approach to fitness is healthy.

PART 1

How Bad Fitness Relationships Take Shape

1

There's No You in Fitness

When you think of the most desirable goals or outcomes in a romantic relationship, what do you think of? True love? Lasting happiness? Does something come to mind?

Even though we often use the word "relationship" in the context of romance, relationships are about how we connect or associate with everything and everyone in our environment. You have a relationship with your friends, kids (if you have them), career, and hobbies, to name a few.

It's nice to wish for the best outcomes with all of these relationships, but sometimes relationships take unhealthy turns. The highs can be high, but the lows can be low. The "mids" can be feel like a stale waste of time. The reality is that relationships can head in many directions.

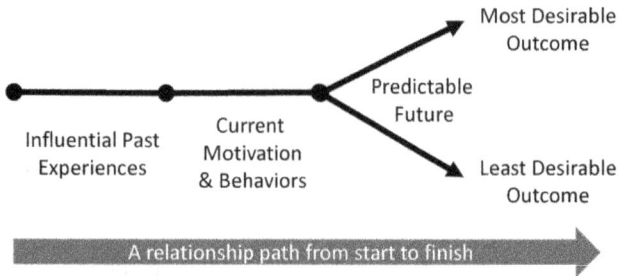

A relationship path from start to finish

Over time, a relationship follows a path that can end up any-where between the most and the least desirable outcomes. This **relationship path**, as I call it, has three parts:

1. **Influential past experiences:** Positive and negative inter-actions and sensory experiences with people, places, and things, including media such as TV, radio, books, podcasts, the internet, advertisements, and more.

2. **Current motivations and behaviors:** Things we want (goals) and don't want, and behaviors that we do and don't do, including repeated habits that have become automatic.

3. **Predictable future:** Our past experiences and present be-haviors set us on a probable trajectory <u>unless we change.</u>

WHERE IS YOUR FITNESS RELATIONSHIP PATH HEADED?

You've had active or passive personal fitness experiences in your past that are related to games, sports, or exercise. Since childhood, you most likely experienced fitness in the context of socially desirable looks and performance goals, like playing and winning in sports. You've seen many fitness ads and have heard about fitness and exercise in the media. Your fitness and exercise past have resulted in feelings and beliefs that are specific to you.

All of this has shaped a fitness path that may not be headed toward maximum health outcomes if you exercise. Alternatively, your past may have steered you away from exercise. Either way, if you think back, you may find that the way you've been conditioned to focus on fitness for looks (e.g. weight loss), performance (e.g. finishing or winning), or social outcomes (e.g. clubs and teams) may not be best for your health. It's not that these outcomes are bad. It's just that many of us don't focus on health as a first priority.

In addition, you may be so emotional about your current fitness path that you are unopen to change. This is what happened to me for years.

I wrote this book to help you discover a health-first fitness path for your body.

Change starts by looking back at how your past influenced your current path, including how some common habits don't help and can hurt joint health, and by questioning if you need a minor or major pivot to address your health. This is Part 2 of the book, after these introductory chapters.

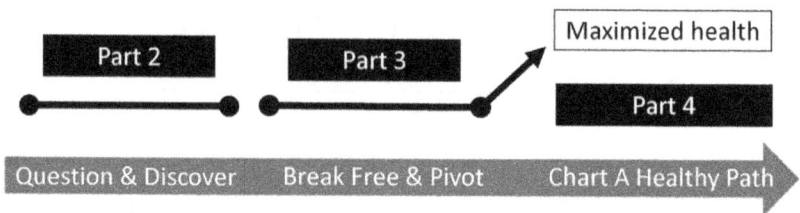

Change continues with a) understanding the fundamentals of bias and habits in order to break free from unhealthy habits and past motivations and b) learning how to build healthy habits. This is Part 3.

And, finally, change involves learning how to set a new course toward better health by becoming aware of your body and defining your starting point. It also involves separating your fitness and weight loss goals to develop a more personalized approach to weight management that considers your unique past and current life factors. This is Part 4.

So why do you need to consider a change? Because it's far too common for fitness paths to not start with a personalized assessment. Yep, it's likely that your fitness path did not consider you.

We often get fitness advice and motivation broadcasted as a one-size-fits-all message to us like this:

"I do this [fitness-or-sport-related thing] which resulted in a looks, performance, or social outcome that I value. Therefore, you should want and do the same. Seriously, you should want and do what I do, to get results that I got, which really matter to me!"

Sound familiar?

Fitness advertising typically operates in this broadcast mode.

They make claims that a certain gadget or workout is the solution for everyone. It's also how many people, including myself for decades, talk to friends, family, and coworkers. We have good intentions and want to share things that we care about. The intent isn't always bad or wrong. Except…

Your body and your starting point are unique and include:

- Your strengths

- Your weaknesses

- Your variances in strength, mobility, or limb length on your left versus right sides

- Your stable or unstable joints

- Your weight

- Your weight distribution

- Your height and height distribution (e.g. you may have longer legs or a longer torso)

- Your past injuries and their impact on your muscles and joints

- How much you sweat

- Your cardiovascular system and conditioning

- Your physiology

- Your health, from your metabolism to mental health issues, like anxiety and depression

- Your lifestyle, including sleep and stress

- Your genetics and how that relates to your ability to perform a specific exercise or sport

- Your fitness past and how that does or doesn't make you feel about exercise

- Your form when you do exercises, including "simple" things like walking and running

All of these things, which are largely silent in fitness marketing and often ignored in fitness culture, impact what happens to your body when you exercise, the odds of your getting specific results from fitness, how long your progress will take, and ultimately, how you feel emotionally or physically about fitness.

This is important. The strength, stability, and mobility of your joints from head to toe determine if and how much positive or negative health gains or losses you will get from your time exercising. But we don't hear this when we get the rah-rah motivation to move.

The fitness brand that's telling you to walk 10,000 steps doesn't know your specific body and health issues. The advertiser doesn't know that weakness or instability in the ankles, knees, or hips may make walking painful for you, as it did for me.

The friend who tells you to run a 10K or marathon doesn't always tell you that running can result in health issues from the feet to the neck.

The friend who suggests yoga may not know that physical therapy should be your first stop to correct any issues and that yoga may never correct them.

The magazine writer who tells you to do a workout to get "long and lean" arms doesn't account for how your genetics—things like limb length and other factors—may make that result less likely or even impossible.

The company or magazine that promotes a six-pack in 30 days does not mention that exercise may have zero impact on your weight loss, depending on other factors. You may need to address things like stress, sleep, emotional or mental health issues, like anxiety or depression—all of which can drive poor eating habits.

The person who says there's "no excuse" for not working out doesn't understand your commute, family responsibilities, work schedule, or finances that changes the calculus of getting to the gym for you.

Many of our cultural fitness goals fail to consider our body, health, abilities, and life factors as the starting point for the exercises we do. Instead, we start our fitness journey based on what others want us to do and without asking ourselves a basic question:

Why do I want good health?

More specifically, we often don't ask ourselves what we care about most in our lives and how improving and maintaining health with fitness can make a difference.

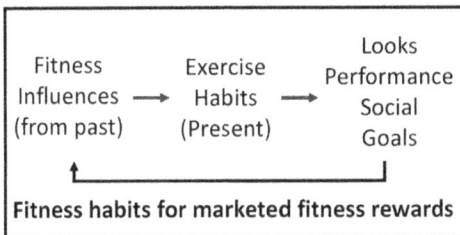

Fitness Influences (from past) $\longrightarrow$	Exercise Habits (Present) $\longrightarrow$	Looks Performance Social Goals	What I love to do now. Who I love to be with. What I want to do for life.
Fitness habits for marketed fitness rewards			**Why I want health**

I'm here to tell you that taking care of your health and body doesn't fit a cookie-cutter script. We wouldn't follow a one-size-fits-all approach for our personal relationships or careers, yet we do it for fitness all of the time.

When you look at your fitness path through the lens of health from start to finish (in other words, for the rest of your life), you may find that your fitness motivation and habits lack:

- A long-term perspective. It's not standard for people, particularly younger people, to think 5 or 10 years out (or longer) about their fitness goals.

- A holistic approach. You may not have thought about your whole health and what you do to take care of it as a measurable, prioritized outcome or goal.

Walking a certain number of steps, finishing a race, or lifting a certain amount of weight are all measurable goals. But the more important holistic goals of good health don't have a standard, widely accepted method to measure it.

By holistic, I mean not just cardiovascular health and other exercise benefits, but long-term, head-to-toe musculoskeletal health. It's possible for everyone to become body aware and understand their own physical strengths, weaknesses, imbalances, and limitations, but there's no standard for this to happen in all fitness settings, even for people who hire personal trainers.

Many of us just jump in without knowing which exercises pose risks given the weaknesses in our body and which exercise are best to correct those weaknesses.

There's a big reason why joint health isn't discussed as a widespread, standard fitness goal. It is among the least talked about and valued part of our fitness past, especially when we were young. We played games, talked about winning, admired pro athletes, and learned exercises to make us stronger or more attractive. Most of us didn't talk about exercising for joint stability and mobility as young men and women. Nor did we see advertisements about the benefits of perfect posture or mobile hips. Unfortunately, this lack of exposure to fitness as a means of holistic health can put us on unhealthy fitness paths early in life.

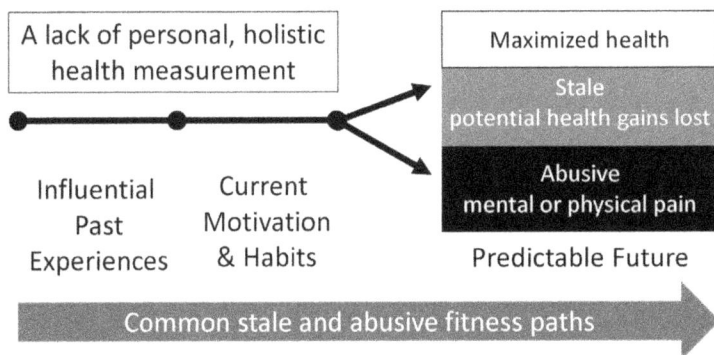

A lack of personal, holistic health measurement

Maximized health

Stale potential health gains lost

Abusive mental or physical pain

Influential Past Experiences

Current Motivation & Habits

Predictable Future

Common stale and abusive fitness paths

When your personal realities are not factored into your fitness choices, your path can track toward common fitness outcomes that don't maximize your health through exercise. They include:

- A stale fitness path, which is exactly like a stale romantic relationship—one where things aren't horrible but for which some meaningful, personal conversations and changes can yield a healthier, more enjoyable life. Tens of millions of people spend thousands of hours exercising without having their strengths and weaknesses assessed holistically. This makes corrections unlikely.

- A physically abusive path, where fitness is the main or contributing cause of degraded joint health or injury.

- A mentally abusive path, where people are: 1) obsessed about looks or performance at the expense of health, including obsessions about diets or 2) alienated, confused, or dispirited by an industry that can be unwelcoming and unsupportive to beginners and those who are unenthusiastic about sport, competition, or fitness extremes.

Far too many of us are on stale and abusive path trajectories that have emotional roots in the experiences of our past. That's why this book is different. I'm here to show you how to change course to build a health-first mindset and program after coming to terms with the influences of your fitness past. It's doable if you're truly open to discovering the degree to which marketing and culture steered your motivation and habits away from health. It's doable if you learn how to become aware of your body, focus on measuring health as your first fitness priority, and then choose the best diversified workout at your level, for your body.

2

How Marketing and Culture Obscure Health

I n my fitness past, I overlooked some obvious warning signs point-
ing to health troubles. In my thirties and early forties, I sometimes
woke up in the morning to find one of my left-hand fingers locked
in a bent "trigger finger" position. I had numbness in my right arm
and pain in my neck.

If I brought my left knee toward my hip, my hip would pop so
loudly people could hear it 20 feet away. My knees would stiffen up
on my ride home from the Saturday morning cycling classes that I
taught. Sometimes I needed to pull myself out of my car. Cycling
was terrible for both my knees and hips[4] [5] [6]given the state of my
body, even though it is advertised as low impact and good for both.
Some of my problems were caused by my personal training sessions
that involved boxing.

I knew my exercise regimen was hurting my body as early as
age 33. But I didn't change until another decade had passed. That's
10 years of ignoring clear warning signs. I ignored them because I
believed I got something out of fitness. I liked teaching hard classes,
doing difficult workouts, and doing things like lifting the entire

stack of weight plates on some machines at my gym. These things were, confoundingly, more important to me than my health.

When I began to consider ending my teaching and boxing training sessions at the same time, my wife and I were both concerned. Those were two things—outside of my relationship with her and our families—that made me happy. It made me think about how crazy it was that things that I knew actually hurt my body made me feel good.

It all ended in 2014 when my wife and I were on our honeymoon in Paris. Though it was the best week of my life, all the walking we did around the city left me with knee and hip pain. I believed I was fit, yet I couldn't walk without feeling pain. How delusional can one person be!?! It was a sobering experience.

I wanted many more decades of strolls with my wife, so after our honeymoon, I decided to divorce fitness as I knew it. I quit all the exercises that I previously did. I was committed to starting over, beginning with doing lots of research on anatomy and corrective exercise strategies for the injured and limited parts of my body.

After a few years had passed, my body felt better than it ever had. It made me ask, why did I stick with a fitness program for so long when I knew it was hurting my body?

Like so many others, I wore fitness blinders.

We simply don't question the health of our fitness path, whether it's people like me who are in pain or people who do the same workout for years without getting assessed.

When I took my blinders off, I realized that I chose that path because many people like me:

- Let the industry define what we want out of fitness. I wanted to be able to do hard workouts and have an athletic build.

- Let the industry captivate us with extreme looks and enviable performance standards. I remember being influenced by movie stars like Sylvester Stallone and Jean-Claude Van Damme and athletes like Walter Payton and Michael Jordan.

- Let the industry tell us that "checking the box" is all we need. I exceeded the government's physical activity guidelines[7] and walked way more than 10,000 steps a day in Paris. Still, a broken body was the result.

- Keep turning to fitness for health, regardless of the fact that weight gain[8] and joint health care expenditures[9] have risen with an increase in exercise over the last 50 years. Not only was I hurting my joints, but I gained weight in my forties despite maintaining a steady workout program.

In other words, we let the fitness industry define what we want out of fitness and it's not always about health.

We've learned to measure "being fit" in two ways: Looks and performance. For many people, that's it. The leaner you are, the harder exercise you do, the fitter you are.

In our culture, it's logical to equate things like:

Lean = Fit
Performance/Athletic Ability = Fit

Believing this logic isn't necessarily a problem. Where this can push a fitness path toward undesirable health outcomes is when we equate this standard of being fit with being healthy. Many if not most of us do that when we assume:

Lean = Fit = Healthy

Performance/Athletic Ability = Fit = Healthy

We assume since our friend ran a marathon, he/she must be healthy, or our coworker or our kid looks great and does fitness competitions or plays sports so he/she must be healthy.

This may or may not be true when we get out of the realm of generalities and shift the conversation to holistic, long-term health. It's also fair to question these assumptions when lean or super-athletic people harbor obsessions or addictions about exercise; those are two common things among fitness enthusiasts that can't be rationalized as being healthy.

The logic of equating looks and performance to health is accentuated by the advertising world. We see people with great bodies scaling walls and participating in running events with the word health next to them. But that's evidence of an ability to do a hard exercise. It's not a measure of health.

If you start measuring health holistically, including head-to-toe joint health, you may need to change a little or a lot in the name of your health. But this can be hard as I learned. The reason is:

We let the industry captivate us with extreme looks and performance standards that we value (emotionally).

Extreme images of models on fitness magazines and product covers have become the benchmark for success. But if we peel back the onion to focus on health, a different story emerges.

The bodies of fitness models in marketing campaigns often have absurdly low body fat. In fact, body builders and fitness competitors are often on the verge of having basic survival levels of body fat. Their body fat levels—often at unhealthy percentages below 12%

for women and 7% for men[10]—are much lower than what the American Council on Exercise calls the "fitness range"—21% to 24% body fat for women and 14% to 27% for men.[11]

Competitors also often take drugs called diuretics to eliminate water in order to show more muscle definition. Yes, in case you didn't know, purposeful dehydration is common in fitness competitions.[12] These same tactics are used by some models in fitness product and magazine shoots.[13] [14]

Then there are stories galore about how participants "pig out" after competitions. Binging is common hours after the photo is taken. Translation: these models don't maintain their cover looks for very long.[15] [16]

Starve. Dehydrate. Brink of survival levels of fat. Pig out. Is this healthy? No way.

Do these images define the cultural standard of "being fit" to which we strive?

Yes! They! Do!

But there's more. The photographs of fitness models are often digitally doctored and aesthetically enhanced in magazines and cover spreads.

Do you see how we can be steered away from thinking about our health? We accept dehydration and airbrushing as the embodiment of being fit and compare ourselves to unattainable images of physical fitness that may not, in fact, represent good health.

Guess what happens when most of us compare ourselves to a leaner model that has been inhumanly airbrushed or unhealthily dehydrated? We lose. Even already lean people can be made to feel bad.

You are likely not surprised that the outside world is a source of envy. You may be surprised to realize how these external influences drive irrational behaviors and biases. Social comparison bias is one of many well-studied cognitive shortcuts that shows the emotional and illogical responses that happen when we compare ourselves to others.

Consider this behavioral science study that asked a group of people the following question—would you rather a) earn $50,000 a year while others earn $25,000 or b) earn $100,000 a year while others earn $200,000? Half, yes half, chose the $50,000 option A, passing on doubling their income in order to be relatively better off than others.[17] [18] Another study showed that bronze medalists are much happier than silver medalists.[19] The bronze winners compare to no medal. The silvers compare to the "what if" of gold.

When looking at the influence of your fitness past on your current motivation and beliefs, it's important to realize that:

- We are innately wired to value achievement relative to others;

  and

- Advertising plays a HUGE role in setting the comparative cultural reference points.

The more people feel far off from the advertised standard, the more impact ads have in triggering a compare-and-lose deficiency that gets our primal brain's attention. They do this with powerful words and sounds but heavily rely on attention-grabbing visuals.

Vision is our most powerful sense. It's hearing for bats, smell for bears, and sight for humans. The visual power of advertising is a big reason why fitness ads featuring extreme bodies and accomplishments have such an influence on our motivation.

We see. We compare. We covet. We see more. We compare again. We covet again. Fitness industry marketing keeps our brains in a perpetual compare-and-lose mode, whether we are young or old, male or female. It takes advantage of our vulnerabilities and makes us feel deficient while making bold, broadcasted promises about how we can change, regardless of our individual starting points. The fitness industry is not alone in selling extreme archetypes. However, other industries, like the fashion industry, don't attach the word health to their products. This is a big difference.

The influence of this extreme standard is creeping in at lower ages than ever before. More than half of girls and a third of boys as young as kindergarten through second grade believe their ideal body should be thinner.[20] [21] These feelings are driven in part by fitness ads and perhaps by always-dieting or always-obsessing-about-being-fat parents who were influenced, in part, by the fitness industry.

It starts young but it can last long. I know men in their fifties who look great, who mention a need to lose five pounds every time I see them.

The pursuit of these standards can negatively impact health. Ultra-physical stress from fitness is possible. Some people can work out so hard, so often, that they can increase stress on the central nervous system. I had the highest frequency of illness like colds and flu when I exercised the most, in my early thirties, at the height of my teaching.

Nutrition can even become a source of unhealthy stress, anxiety, and obsession when linked to weight. Psychologists have coined the term orthorexia nervosa, a condition where people take eating healthy to obsessive levels.[22] There seems to be obsession all around us with people who are on extreme, all-or-nothing diets.

I know someone who left a dinner with friends to exercise because they felt they ate too much. "Exercise bulimia"[23] [24] is a term coined by psychology experts to describe a condition that involves purging with exercise instead of throwing up. However, if we looked at these people, many of us would call them fit and healthy solely based on how they look.

We also let the fitness industry tell us that "checking the box" is all we need to do to be fit and healthy.

Walk 10,000 steps every day. Set your watch or phone to alert you to stand every hour. Lift weights twice per week. Do cardio three times a week. Do yoga.

That's activity tracking. That's not customized measurement and tracking of the health of your body. Yet many of us presume health when we check a box.

Similarly, the industry, fitness experts, and even friends make health claims all the time.

This class or fad is healthy.

That exercise is healthier.

These exercises are better than those.

Most of these claims are not coupled with a way to objectively measure health.

Measuring health holistically with a proactive, culturally approved, and standard method simply doesn't exist, particularly when you include head-to-toe joint health.

Since the early 1970s, about the time when modern fitness was born, the fitness and fitness apparel industries have made trillions of dollars. Sales in health club memberships, health and fitness magazines, and at-home fitness equipment and machines have all soared since then. There is simply no doubt that the number of people who exercise has soared in 50 years. For example, 55 people ran the New York City marathon in 1970[25] compared to 52,000 in 2019.[26] And yet, over the same period, health issues like diabetes, obesity, and joint issues have also risen.[27] [28] [29] [30] [31] [32] [33]

I'm not saying that fitness is always unhealthy or the sole cause of these epidemics.

I am making these assertions:

- We need to challenge the industry's claims that exercise plays a primary role in weight loss when many people use their machines, do their programs, and check their boxes but still don't lose weight.

- We need to accept that making a general statement that "exercise is healthy" without factoring in joint health, and directing people how to measure it, is incomplete at best.

- We need to recognize that the fitness industry influences our motivation and goals with extreme, aspirational images of fitness instead of directing us what works best for our personal realities and our health.

You know another industry that boosted esteem and talked about health in their marketing but kept people in the dark about health warnings? The tobacco industry. Like the fitness industry, it spent a lot of time and advertising dollars to impart social value to their products.

Cigarette ads conveyed a sense of bravado, manliness, and success for men. Women were targeted with the "torches of freedom" campaign to link smoking to women's equality and independence.

Just like fitness ads, cigarette ads promoted health, from weight loss to dental health and (unbelievably) asthma relief.[34] [35] [36] [37]

Despite the 1964 Surgeon General's warning[38] about the dangers of smoking, researchers showed that "in the mid-1960s it was still common to see doctors, athletes, and radio, movie, and TV celebrities smoking or advertising different cigarette brands, and cigarette companies were major sponsors of popular shows on all three television networks." Yes.[39] [40] Doctors were on that list.

The decline in cigarette smoking can be traced to widespread public warnings and a ban on TV and radio cigarette ads that started in 1970, after the *Public Health Cigarette Smoking Act* of 1969.[41] At this same time in history, fitness, sports, and fitness apparel industries began their 50-year marketing campaign that mirrored the tobacco industry.

It can take years for the impact of our habits, whether related to smoking or fitness, to catch up with us. But it's never too late to change. And that change starts with your openness to questioning your fitness motivation and habits.

3

Tuning in to Your Body and Mind

After I divorced fitness, for the first time in my life I felt like I didn't know how to exercise. I knew I wanted good health, but I didn't know where to turn.

I did, however, know where *not* to turn. I was done with the delusion that "feeling good" from exercising was an indicator of health. I felt great teaching and from being able to do hard workouts. All that "feeling good" resulted in a broken body.

I also understand from personal experience that knowing a lot about fitness or exercise isn't the answer either. Knowing how to exercise for looks or performance is not the same as knowing how to assess the function of a body and correct problems.

I knew that exercising for cardiovascular health is powerful, and it's easy to get tested by doctors at insurance-approved, annual checkups for those with insurance. They have standard tests that are used from coast to coast. Equally important, there are easily understood scores for health indicators like blood pressure. It's easy to find out with well-established benchmarks if your blood pressure is good, bad, or somewhere in between.

This is great. Half of American adults have some form of cardiovascular disease.[42] It can kill. We need to be on the lookout for any related cardiovascular red flags. But what about a heads up for things like musculoskeletal issues that can limit your function and make life miserable? Half of American adults have these issues, which impact quality of life.

I know a senior executive with enhanced insurance who gets an annual medical exam that includes a bone density scan and stress test. Just like at my annual checkup, the doctor doesn't spend any time assessing joint health. In fact, my experience was that many therapists and doctors who do the best head-to-toe musculoskeletal assessments (and they are not easy to find) do not take insurance. Their fees typically range from $120 to $250 per hour, out of pocket. One therapist quoted a six-session minimum for $1,000 before providing treatment.

Half of American adults have clinical, musculoskeletal issues and many people have preclinical musculoskeletal symptoms in the form of tightness or muscle imbalance. Still, no affordable, standard, and proactive process exists to diagnose and correct head-to-toe musculoskeletal health, or structural health, as I prefer to call it.

"Structural health" is a term I use to describe the strength, stability, range of motion, left-to-right balance (symmetry), and alignment of our muscles, joints, soft tissue, and bones—the underlying structure of our bodies. I prefer the term structural health over the medical and antiseptic-sounding word musculoskeletal health. This preference is driven by how clinical and unapproachable I found joint research to be for the general population.

Exercise is an untapped, affordable solution to many structural health issues if you are aware of your body and prioritize corrective exercises. But structural health may not be on your radar. I had tons of positive fitness experiences in my life, but this topic was simply never front and center, if it was even mentioned at all.

Structural health never came up in any departmental meeting at any gym where I taught. It never came up in the thousands of group exercise classes that I've taken. I never saw an advertisement for a product or activity that directed me to get my structural health assessed before I started a fitness routine. In fact, my walking gait and posture were so obviously dysfunctional that someone could have noticed the problem from 50 feet away. Not one person mentioned it in any of the 10 gyms where I worked.

I know more about structural health now than when I was a fitness instructor because of the extensive research I've done to regain my health. It's also because I was hell-bent on going to numerous structural health therapists, all of whom taught me something different and valuable about my body.

The reality is that there are varying degrees of knowledge of structural health in the fitness industry. You may find a great personal trainer or instructor who knows how to assess your body. You may find someone in the industry who talks about joint mobility and stability as a prerequisite to exercise in a particular way.

They're out there. And they're invaluable.

Some personal trainers, however, start a conversation with "What do you want to work on?" or "What are your fitness goals?" Those questions usually relate to looks- or performance-related goals. How can anyone pursue a structural health-related goal if no one tells them why stable and mobile joints matter? And that's just individuals who hire a personal trainer. Most people who work out in health clubs or exercise independently don't even get that.

We simply start exercising with no assessment of our body, or our level, for that matter.

If someone walked into a martial arts studio and said they wanted to be a black belt in six months, they would likely be asked to leave. Martial arts programs mandate advancement in a predetermined method based on qualifications.

There is no such "belt system" for advancement in all areas of fitness. For example, if someone wanted to run a marathon or 10K in six months, they may not have anyone who checks to see if running is an appropriate or safe activity for their body, now or in the future. The same is true for many areas in fitness: Olympic lifting, kettlebells, whatever. You may find a place that has its own standards and provides level advancement and coaching. You may not. There just aren't universal standards and there should be.

When classes are offered at different levels, some people prefer to trudge through a higher-level class with horrible form versus putting in the time to learn proper form at a lower level. I saw this often as an instructor. Many people just want to jump in and go as fast and as hard as they can.

If health is your priority, your path needs to begin with defining it holistically, which means taking into account your structural health. But structural health is just one part of health.

So what is a healthy fitness relationship path that considers health holistically? There's no simple answer to this question, but I can show you the elements that lead you there.

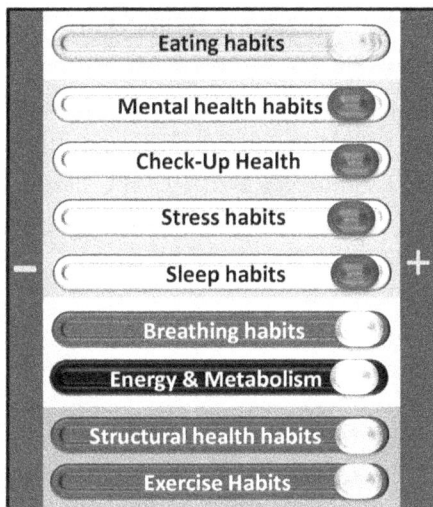

Fitness Health Tuner

I'd like to introduce you to the fitness health tuner, which is how I learned to divide and conquer the ways I reclaimed my health after my fitness divorce. I learned that I needed to understand all of these things individually if I was going to improve my health, and I studied and improved on each of them over the past six years.

Why is it important to include all of these elements? It's important because you want to fine tune different aspects of your health in different ways, depending on your unique, personal factors. You also don't want to focus on goals like weight loss to the exclusion of other goals, such as structural health.

Eating habits are far and away the most important factor in weight loss and management. But the term "diet" is often discussed in a vacuum. In fact, four other elements (shown in white in the diagram above) besides diet also can significantly impact eating habits.

I call these four elements—checkup health, stress, sleep, and mental health—the "Silent 4" that never come up when we hear about weight loss promises in fitness ads and the never-ending "diet and exercise" weight loss narrative. However, addressing any one or several of these four tuning levels may be the most important bridge to cross for some people in achieving lasting weight management habits. They're all related.

Why? It's because many people eat poorly as a habitual reaction to stress, depression, anxiety, anger, sadness, or another negative state of mind. Bad sleep habits too, can translate into more eating and less exercising due to low energy.

Despite the numerous benefits of exercise, it's absurd to talk about exercise as a weight loss savior or diet in terms of things to eat and not eat, while ignoring the influence of our unique past experiences and how they've impacted our "Silent 4" tuning levels. We can't just "go on a diet" and expect emotional and psychological habits to go away after they've been hardwired into our neurological system over a lifetime.

I know because I had to learn how to tune my Silent 4 to lose weight. Regular exercise didn't make a dent, even though I regularly exercised and burned a lot of calories in every workout.

Now that you've seen the nine levels in the tuner, you may be asking: what is tuning?

Tuning is about learning and accepting where you are and embracing incremental, gradual gains from your starting point. It's aimed at eliminating the all-or-nothing focus of fitness, particularly for weight loss and performance goals. It's about building lasting habits in all areas of life that advance health holistically. These improvements can be measured in different ways, qualitatively or quantitatively.

For example, sleep hours can be counted or measured by devices like smartphones, apps, or with professionally administered tests. Eating can be with an app or you can do estimated tracking in your head. You can set heart rate targets with age-based charts[43] [44]or, more elaborately, with VO2 max tests.

You can measure structural health with the assistance of therapists who test your muscles and joints. Exercises can be used, too, as general indicators of your ability to control and stabilize certain movements with specific parts of your body.

In any case, tuning is about measuring and tracking health in small increments so that you can celebrate small wins while you gradually build lasting habits. It's about dividing and conquering the things that impact your health the most, starting with how you are tuned in each level right now. This is the starting point that needs to be gauged before setting your fitness and weight loss goals.

To help you understand tuning, imagine that you started watching eight shows on a streaming service like Netflix or Hulu but didn't finish any of them. You stopped after a certain number of episodes or midway through one. When you log in to resume watching, your television or computer saved where you left off.

How does this relate to fitness? Your starting point for each tuning level is based on your past, including your genetics. Fitness intersects with each aspect of your health and your habits in different ways.

Once you know your starting point, you can choose what to work on first in the tuner, just like you can decide which show to resume. Working on one thing at a time versus trying to do everything at once improves your chances of building enduring habits and improving your health.

We'll cover the tuner more in-depth in the final part of the book. I'm introducing it here for two reasons.

First, just like financial returns on investments of money, getting the most returns out of time invested in fitness varies. When I talk about maximizing health outcomes with your time exercising throughout this book, I'm defining this as tuning as many levels as positively as possible, staring with where you are in each.

Second, it's important to know what holistic health and productive tuning looks like before you assess how your past has influenced health on your fitness path. There are three types of tuning, including:

- Healthy tuning is when you maximize your progress at every level.

- Stale tuning is when you are stuck because you haven't figured out how to personally measure, track, and tune habits at each level.

- Abusive tuning is when you have habits that negatively impact your health in one or more levels in the short or long term.

For many years, I used exercise to positively tune several of my levels, including checkup health, metabolism, and self-esteem (mental health). But my structural health went in the negative direction. I never took the time to address bad eating habits along with sleep and stress issues, which played a big role in my bad eating habits for years. That's a textbook definition of abusive tuning.

Now that you have an idea on how to define a healthy fitness path with holistic health tuning, it's time for an honest, introspective look at how your fitness past has influenced your fitness motivation, priorities, and health.

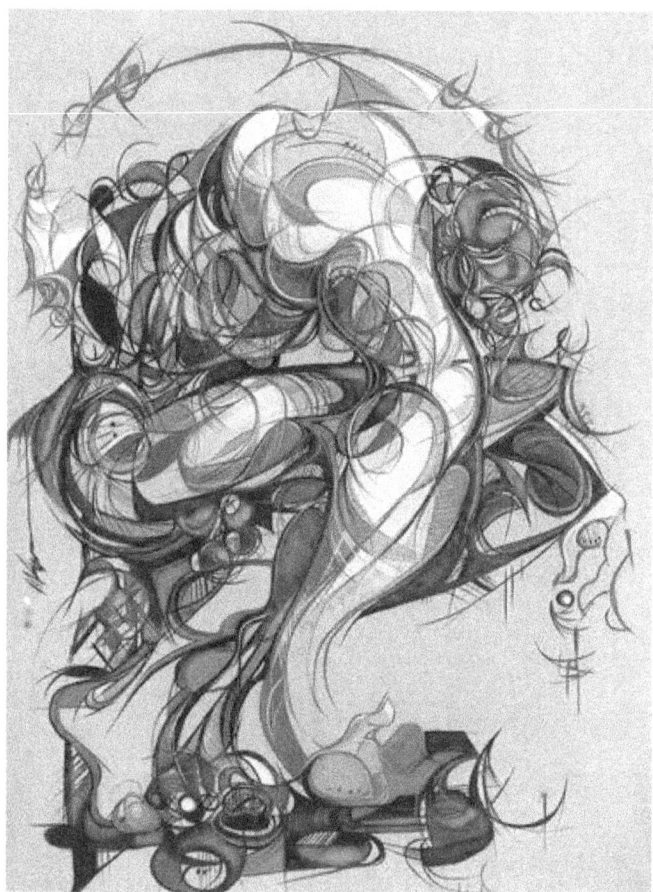

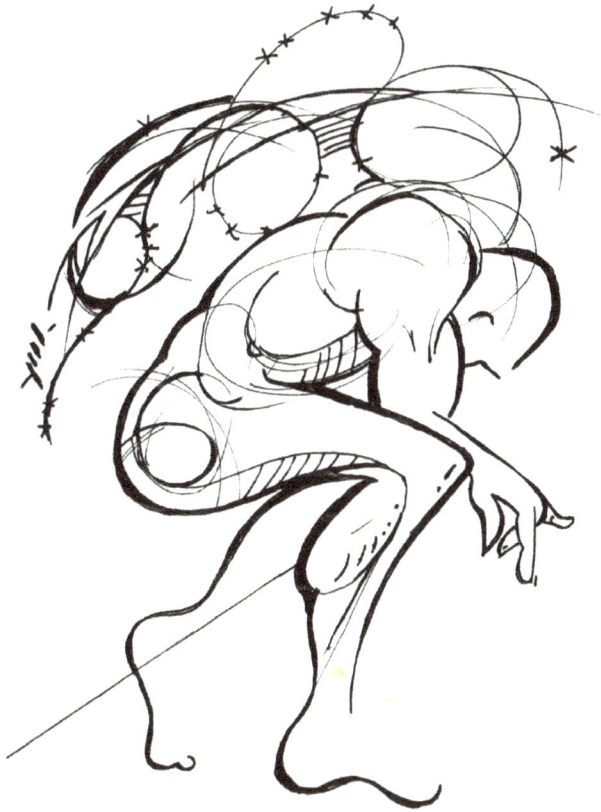

PART 2

Your Fitness Past –
Where is It Leading You?

W hen I saw the first drawing on the previous page for the first
time, I saw the power of the human body trapped in pain.
It takes effort to realize that the subject of the drawing on the left is
the same man in the drawing on the right. I found that health was
equally unclear and abstract in fitness.

The following chapters are about discovering what your fitness
past taught you to want and value. Specifically, how do your actions
or goals—which represent what you value—for looks, performance,
or social outcomes align with the goal of measuring and tracking
good health holistically?

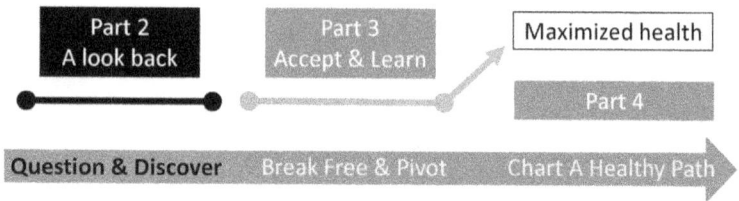

Each chapter will allow you to answer questions on how your past experiences with fitness industry marketing and culture have influenced you. When people go to therapy to change, they often start by learning and accepting the roots of their current behaviors.

4

Are You Ignoring
Your Body?

In personal relationships, it's often the little things that keep people happy, from being reliable and considerate of someone's time to being grateful and courteous. These traits, while they may be boring to put on a dating wish list, are foundational to healthy relationships.

Unfortunately, there are some equally "boring" topics that relate to how your body works that matter to your health and fitness. I didn't recognize their importance until I went paddle boarding for the first time.

Two years into my fitness divorce, my wife called me. She was excited. She had just bought paddle boarding lessons after getting a coupon via email. We went down to Montrose Beach in Chicago on a beautiful summer day, excited to try it for the first time.

I stood up on the board effortlessly. By this time, I had built up core strength after a few years of Pilates, yoga, and physical therapy. I was cruising. Balance was easy for the first five minutes, then I felt the board wobble.

Splash. I got back up. The wobbling got worse as I overcorrected.

I tried unsuccessfully a few more times. I was frustrated. I didn't know why but all of a sudden, my body couldn't do something that was effortless a few minutes ago.

The next few times on the board, I felt heavy cramping in my outer left ankle and high up my inner left thigh near the groin. It got so bad I couldn't stand. My paddle boarding career ended before it started. Frustrated, I swam back to shore.

My wife, meanwhile, paddle boarded out from the placid marina to the choppier waters of Lake Michigan and did great.

I had a big health revelation after paddle boarding. My left ankle was really weak and unstable, even though it didn't hurt. In fact, I didn't have any symptoms of ankle pain for decades, though I broke it and suffered ligament damage when I was 15 years old. I also had lots of ankle sprains from sports in my latter teens and early twenties.

Paddle boarding is an activity that requires the left and right legs to work equally. If they are imbalanced in strength or stability, a stronger leg will push down onto the board more than a weaker leg. And then the wobbling starts.

This experience illuminated not just the weak links in my body, it also showed me how one compromised part in the body impacts everything else. My ankle and hip were weak when trying to work together.

Discovering the connection between my left hip and left ankle was one of the most important health insights of my life. It happened because I tried something new. It happened because my wife opened an unsolicited marketing email.

It's a story that serves as an intro to the goal of this chapter, which is answering this question: How many of the following **Unmarketed topics** have you heard of and factored into your fitness choices and priorities? These topics simply don't come up regularly in fitness marketing and cultural conversations. But they really matter.

So, are you ignoring these **Unmarketed topics** in general and when making your fitness choices?

Unmarketed topic 1: Most of us aren't operating with factory default settings.

We have factory default settings on our phones and car radios. Who changes them? We do. Why? In response to the way we uniquely use them.

The body has defaults as well. Each of our muscles has a specific purpose. Each has a default length. Each of our 600-plus muscles has a default level of strength and an optimal ratio of strength and mobility relative to other muscles with which it works. Muscles initiate, control, and stabilize movement and balance. Muscles attach to bones through what are called tendons. Muscles can get shorter. We know this as tightness. Muscles can get longer or weaker.

Bones support the body, resisting gravity, and work with muscles to move. They have default alignment relative to other bones. A joint is where two bones meet for the purpose of movement. Different joints have varying degrees of movement. They are designed to work with specific muscles to move in different directions. Default range and mobility of joints can change. An example of this is not being able to bend and come close to touching your toes.

Your defaults in muscles, bones, or soft tissue can change in a way that is unique to you. For some people, it may just be a little. But for half of us, the changes lead to a musculoskeletal disorder. Your past influences how your defaults get changed.

What causes defaults to change? A past injury is a big reason, particularly when someone doesn't do a full course of physical therapy. I didn't do therapy after my ankle breaks and sprains, and the defaults changed. A lot! But it's not just injuries that alter defaults.

Unmarketed topic 2: Everyday life alters our defaults.

Lots of things in modern life negatively alter our structural health defaults, whether it's being right- or left-handed, excessive computer mouse use, crossed legs, carrying a bag or backpack, and smartphone use. Things like "texting thumb," caused by tendon inflammation in tendon, can result from single-side overuse.[45]

Shoes also can change structural health defaults. Heels alter your natural hip alignment, which changes the muscles used to control your feet, ankles, knees, and hips while walking.[46] Shoes can also change the way we use foot and toe muscles.

The instability of my outer left ankle led me to walk on the outside of my foot for years. This limited the use of my big toe from using its full range of motion. I figured out why this mattered after my paddle boarding experience when I read online that "the great toe joint can be linked to compensation patterns ranging from over-recruitment of the adductors (inner thighs) to inhibition of the gluteus maximus."[47] [48] Translation: Not using my big toe as designed made my inner thighs work in overdrive for years, while my left butt muscles were working differently than the right. Yep. The big toe is a big deal. How we use it impacts how muscles get used up the body.

Modern life impacts our defaults in other ways. Walking on even surfaces limits the number of ways we use our feet and ankles. Modern toilets limit range as well. By not getting into the deep squat used by our ancestors and people in Eastern cultures to this day, we limit the range of muscles used in the ankles, knees, hips, and spine.

The same is true for our shoulders, our most mobile joints. People who only do cardio like running or walking may rarely use their arms overhead. In most jobs, it's not a requirement to lift our arms that way. We aren't swinging from trees to survive anymore.

Defaults in joints and muscles change when we don't use joints in all of their natural ranges of motion.

You've heard the expression "use it or lose it." That applies to joint range of motion.

A huge crusher of structural health is—drum roll, please—sitting. Sitting can alter defaults and how the top and middle of the body[49] [50] are balanced.

The only thing worse than sitting is sitting while looking at screens because we've become a nation of slouchers. People have coined the term "text neck" for the damage to the upper body and neck caused by our overuse of devices. It's a problem starting at younger and younger ages.[51] [52]

When you aren't aware of your specific default changes, you may be exercising with limitations or weaknesses. I call any such limitations "weak links," and they can range from major, diagnosable health issues to simple tightness.

I learned an important lesson while paddle boarding, which is that the saying "you are as strong as your weakest link" rings powerfully true for the human body.

Unmarked topic 3: Parts are not programmed to work alone. The have chained, interdependent default requirements.

Engineers don't design parts of a car in separate rooms before figuring out the entire car. The tires work with the shocks, which work with the suspension system, which works with the steering system, and so on. An optimal performing car has "chained" parts that co-operate with other parts.

That's how the body is designed to work. But fitness culture doesn't always talk about chained interdependence of parts and instead often focuses on only one part of the body in isolation—for example, we are told that crunches are a great ab exercise or squats work your butt.

I'd like you to think about exercises as using multiple muscles across a chain of interconnected joints to control and stabilize body movement through a specific range of motion.

I know. That's a little bit technical. But it's important to understand, so let's break it down.

When you can do an exercise through a full range with proper form, without wobbling or misalignment, you:

- Have strength in the dominant muscles to control and stabilize the movement.

- Have enough strength in the supportive, nondominant muscles to control and stabilize the movement.

- Have enough mobility in the muscles and joints to move without restriction.

Let's take a squat as an example. The *support* muscles for this exercise are the spinal erectors, abs, hamstrings, calves, and smaller butt muscles like the gluteus medius and minimus. You also need a base level of ankle, knee, hip, and back mobility to execute the move. Is that what you think of when you think of a squat? It's natural to think of a squat as a butt or, perhaps, quadriceps (a.k.a. quad) exercise. Those two, plus the inner thighs, are the *dominant* muscles.

This is important to understand: culturally, we tend to talk about exercises in terms of the dominant muscles and not the support players in the chain used for that exercise.

Paddle boarding showed me that I had interconnected weak links when the muscles in my feet tried to work with muscles up through the center of my body. Had I gone to my gym that morning I could have lifted the entire stack of weight on the inner thigh machine with ease. But my inner thigh muscles shut down when they were forced to work with the chain of muscles through my feet. Working parts in isolation doesn't always tell the story.

Of course, take any localized symptoms and pain relief measures seriously. However, it's important to broaden your focus to understanding how the rest of your body comes into play. My hip issues didn't get better, for instance, until I focused on my feet and ankles after the paddle boarding experience.

Also, please be open to the fact that I learned way too late: You may be able to exercise moderately or do high performance workouts—like long runs or be able to lift a lot of weight—and still have some or many minor or major weaknesses and limitations. It may take time for symptoms to manifest.

Do you talk about exercises holistically in terms of how all the parts of your body are working together? Or do you tend to talk about exercises for specific areas? Are you familiar with the concept of the chain, and have you heard about it in fitness? If so, to what degree, and have you had your chain assessed?

Unmarketed topic 4: Left-to-right muscle and joint balance is a big deal.

What if the left tires on your car had 10 pounds less pressure than the right tires? Would you take the family on a road trip without fixing it? What if two legs of your kitchen stool were loose? Would you have a family member sit on it? Hopefully, you answered no to both questions. Still, we exercise with left-to-right imbalances all the time, knowingly or not.

Though "perfect" left-to-right balance, also called symmetry, isn't a must for a healthy life, not attending to a left-to-right muscle or joint imbalance raises the likelihood that it will get worse.

I've heard many fitness instructors say it's normal to have imbalances. I've probably said the same thing. Like them, I never jumped up and down to make big deal about it. Today, though, I know it is a big deal.

Frankly, I consider it to be among the greatest failures of the fitness industry to not drive people to make left-to-right imbalances a top fitness goal.

Has anyone in the fitness industry or the structural health care system assessed your left-to-right symmetry? If so, did they assign corrective exercises, and did you measure and track your progress? Or are you like many who exercise without considering this at all?

Unmarketed topic 5: Front-to-back balance is a big deal.

The front-to-back defaults in our body, which also are important for structural health, are managed by collaborative pairs of muscles such as the biceps and triceps or the quads (thighs) and hamstrings.

These partners are meant to have specific ratios when it comes to front-to-back strength and muscle length. One way our front-to-back defaults get changed in a bad way is when partner muscles lengthen or shorten—in other words, they get tight. This type of imbalance is common in the neck, shoulders, back, and hips but it can be anywhere. Sitting a lot and using electronic devices can play a big role in causing imbalances in the top and middle of the body.

Front-to-back imbalances should be understood and corrected or exercise can make things worse. Most of us know muscle pairs like the biceps and triceps because these are the showy ones that are featured in advertisements and group exercise classes. But learning about the other important parts of the body helps you monitor your weaknesses and overall health.

For instance, can you name the partner of the gluteus maximus, the largest butt muscle, on the front of your body? It's the psoas, which is known as a hip flexor, and it significantly impacts your posture and the stability of your spine.[53] [54] [55] Some experts call it one of the most important muscles in the body.

Can you name the partner set of muscles to your front-facing, six-pack abs? It's a group called the erector spinae, a group of muscles critical for posture and spinal mobility.

These are just two examples that show how our fitness culture and marketing have influenced what we know and care about in terms of our health.

Unmarked topic 6: Physics (including weight) makes the same exercise different for different people.

What do cars, planes, trains, and a human body in motion have in common? They are all mechanical systems with interdependent parts subject to the laws of physics.

A big part of your body's physics is your total mass—namely, the sum total of your bones, fluids, organs, and fat. Body fat is just part of our mass. Some of us have extra mass because of our larger frames or parts.

The more mass you have, the more force you absorb and the more force it takes to move you. Right now, you are absorbing force from the ground, your chair, your bed…whatever is connected to the earth.

During exercise, you absorb more force.

The amount of force is generally determined by your mass (weight), the distance traveled (how far you move), and for how long.

During most exercises like running, walking, or squats, your feet and ankles are the first point of contact to absorb the load. The foot, for example, takes on two to three times your body weight while walking. Multiply your weight by two or three times and that's how much force your knee absorbs when you walk. Multiply your weight by a greater factor of 5 to 12 times to determine the load your knee handles while running.[56] Of course, this all depends on things like form, but now you understand one reason why doctors recommend weight loss for people with issues from the hips down.

As someone who is lean at 245 pounds and has weighed as much as 295, I learned the hard way why we all can't be jockeys. More weight means more forces are absorbed by the body when we exercise.

When he was having symptoms, NBA player Derrick Rose said that he saw numerous doctors who didn't tell him that the few extra pounds he was carrying influenced his knee pain.[57]

Fitness can take an unhealthy turn when total mass (weight) is not considered.

Has anyone ever talked to you about how your body type, including your weight or ratios of limb length, contribute to the efficiency, inefficiency, or risk of certain exercises?

Unmarketed topic 7: Weak links can prevent good exercise form. Bad form can make weak links weaker.

Proper form means that muscles are properly aligned, controlling and stabilizing the body in all ways —from front to back and side to side. Form plays a big role in whether you are or are not maximizing health outcomes with exercise. Along with protecting your structural health, form also impacts how you absorb forces.

Form can even impact professional athletes if it isn't proactively assessed. Lorenzo Cain is an All-Star major league baseball player who had chronic hamstring injuries. Changing his running form saved his career. The way he ran stressed his hamstrings. Since he is a powerful athlete and big guy, more power plus more mass plus bad form forced his hamstrings to take on more load than they could handle. Yes, a professional athlete needed to learn how to run. But no one told him to focus on form during his first few years in the minor and major leagues.[58]

Form also can be compromised when modifications are substituted for proper structural health assessments. Pull-ups are a good example because they're so popular in many fitness circles. An internet search on how to avoid elbow pain while doing pull-ups reveals articles that suggest modifying the exercise by using a band, chair, or machine. But such a modification fails to help someone who doesn't have enough scapular (shoulder blade) or shoulder mobility. In other words, the pull-ups will continue to load the elbow joint in unhealthy ways[59] even if they are doing modifications.

Good form, even when doing simple things like walking, can be impossible with structural health limitations. However, you may not know this in a fitness culture simply lacks a standard to communicate this message, "Before you try this exercise, you should be able to do (a list of required movements that demonstrate the ability to try an exercise with less risk)."

Has anyone assessed your form for the exercises that you do, including walking or running?

Were you informed about how joint immobility, muscle weakness, or joint instability can limit proper form for exercises that you like?

Unmarketed healthy process: Exercise for structure first.

If there is one place that health-first fitness should start, it's with structural health, which includes understanding how our chained defaults are working (or not working) as designed.

Start with structure first, looking for any limitations in strength, stability, mobility, or left-to-right or front-to-back imbalances. If any weak links are identified, small or major, the first priority is to correct them with a physician or professional trainer (or both). Weak links can get even weaker when exercising, if left unattended.

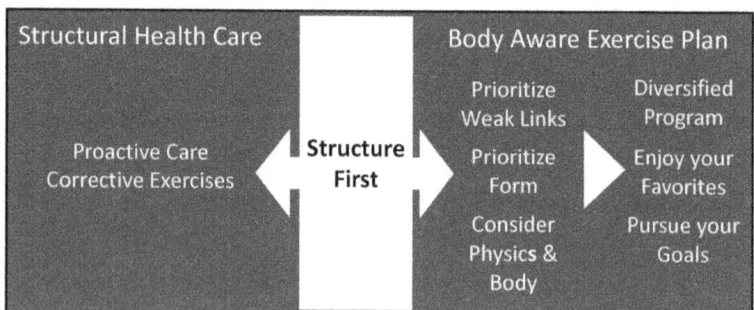

Structural Health Care	Structure First	Body Aware Exercise Plan	
Proactive Care Corrective Exercises		Prioritize Weak Links	Diversified Program
		Prioritize Form	Enjoy your Favorites
		Consider Physics & Body	Pursue your Goals

HEALTH-FIRST FITNESS
PUTS STRUCTURE FIRST

After you've addressed any issues, it's time to consider the match between your body and a specific exercise, like considering your total mass for things like running that favor lighter people with less upper body mass. Then focus on form, especially if you choose workouts like running, sports, or lifting heavy weights. Finally, and only after ensuring that your body is ready for a specific type of exercise, you can pursue your fitness goals and enjoy your favorite exercises or sports.

To be clear, I'm not against any type of exercise. I'm for the equivalent of warnings on cigarette packages, created by people and companies who sell or advocate specific exercises, that communicate how and why specific exercises may not be a good fit for specific bodies. These same people and companies should direct people how and where to test for exercise fit and risks.

This process is not a fad. It's not a gimmick. When you adhere to it, you're maximizing your odds for excellent short- and long-term health. Risk is minimized and performance will be improved for simple activities like walking or running or more demanding workouts, such as power lifting or training for extreme events.

It's also important to understand that the human body is resilient. It's magnificently built to survive. That can keep us moving for decades without experiencing symptoms of developing issues. I only felt symptoms with my ankle when I tried to run. I didn't have a clue that my ankle, my upper back, and core were weak until I tried to balance on a paddleboard.

If you haven't done so while reading this chapter, please reflect on how you were influenced in your fitness past to consider and prioritize your body's:

1.　Function (Structural Health), including weak links and imbalances.

2.　Form, which can create weakness or injury.

3.　Physics, which means your total mass (weight) matters in general and more when structural health and form are compromised.

Were you assessed and taught why this is important to your health before exercising? If so, did you make it a priority or ignore it?

5

Complete Program or "Sexy" Muscle Focus?

Good parents with multiple children don't focus solely on one child. Smart corporations don't just hire sales, operations, and marketing teams without finance, HR, and legal. Top car manufacturers don't establish quality assurance programs for engines and transmissions but not for brakes and the drive train.

Having a limited focus on only specific parts of a complex system like a family, company, or car can yield unhealthy or unsafe results because neglect anywhere impacts the system as a whole.

This also applies to fitness. Too many of us have fallen into our culture's tendency to focus on the "sexy" or "hot" parts of our bodies without taking care of the rest.

This chapter is a look at how ads and culture shaped your motivation to see if you have a holistic focus on health with your exercises, like lifting and strength training, outside of traditional cardio. Or if you've fallen into a cultural tendency to focus on exercises for the "sexy" parts.

To help answer this question, consider the areas you care about the most and what contributed to that focus.

Fitness marketing and culture teach us that being "hot" is a coveted fitness goal. Everywhere. From magazines, programs sold via informercials, equipment, and exercise DVD covers, it's almost guaranteed to bring on the hot body full-court press.

Words like sexy, thin, and perfect are core parts of fitness advertising lingo. There are literally products or magazine article titles with the word "perfect" prominently featured.

The fitness industry uses words like sculpt, cut, and chisel— words associated with a perfectly carved figure—that remind us of ancient marble sculptures. Many ads are sexually explicit, featuring over-thin women with toned arms and ultra-buff men with rippled chests. I saw one ad for a gym with an image of a woman crawling on a pool table in a short cocktail dress to promote a health club.[60]

There's nothing wrong with sex appeal or trying to look attractive. I'm not a prude. What I want to draw your attention to is the fact that the industry often focuses on less than 20 muscles—what I call the "Right Swipe" muscles because they get the most attention in fitness and on dating apps—when our bodies have more than 600. In other words, there are direct correlations between what is advertised, what is known and talked about, and what is prioritized in workouts.

The grand marshal of the hot body parade is the abdomen, especially the front six-pack abs. They are followed by the biceps and triceps, which are often airbrushed in photos for best effect, and sometimes the deltoids. The chest, butt, and quads (thighs) get lots of attention, too, with lunges and squats promoted everywhere you look.

Inner thigh exercises are a good place to look at how ads influence our fitness habits. Inner thigh ads are primarily targeted at women, even though this muscle group is critical to everyone's structural health and plays a major role in healthy walking and running gaits.

Though they may exist, I have not found one man in a fitness ad doing or advocating inner thigh exercises. The inner thigh machine gets used by more women than men in the gyms. Some men don't, or won't, do any inner thigh exercises.

Unfortunately, this is one way that the fitness industry can drive beliefs that an exercise is gendered. There are people who associate certain types of exercises or exercises for certain body parts in this way.

There are others who develop unhealthy and untrue perceptions about certain exercises. After teaching a cycling class, I was approached by a woman who told me that she liked my class but she didn't want to come back because she didn't want her legs to look like mine. I weighed 240 pounds at the time and she probably weighed about 110.

The important lesson is to be open to how your priorities have been influenced in a way that may not be in the best interest of your health. You may be walking away from important exercises because of misconceptions and misinformation, some of which has been influenced by marketing or trusted sources in your past.

Please take a look back and think about what body parts you think of the most when you think of fitness. Are they problem areas in your mind? How many muscles or parts can you name that get your attention in your current or desired program?

It's common to have a list that is limited to the Right Swipes. To be clear, healthy and strong Right Swipes are important. Also, fitness industry marketers did not drive us to be physically attracted to these parts. However, fitness marketing could advertise joint health, but it doesn't happen.

As a result, two problems arise.

The first is that you are assumed to be structurally sound when people tell you about the benefits of an exercise. You may be getting health benefits from an exercise like a squat or dead lift. You may not be. It depends on your form, function, and physics, but no one tells you to get your structural health assessed before jumping in and trying it.

The second problem with this Right Swipe focus is that it prioritizes certain parts of the body while ignoring others that can disrupt your balance and structural health.

To understand this, consider whether any of the following statements apply to you.

I ignore the top of my body. The reality is that modern life can severely impact neck function. And the neck works closely with the shoulders and upper back, including the muscles that connect to the shoulder blade. Excessive sitting leads to forward head posture (FHP)—a condition where the chin (skull) is too far forward, or forward and down, and out of proper vertical alignment. It's often accompanied by slouched shoulders and a rounded upper back. This disrupts front-to-back function at the top of the chain.

Every inch of forward head posture can increase the weight of the head on the spine by an additional 10 pounds.[61] This is a big deal. It's a bigger deal when exercising because we absorb even more force than normal.

Fitness programs can skip lots of muscles and ranges of motion at the top of the body. Exercises like chest stretches, neck and scapular mobility exercises, rotator cuff exercises, Pilates "swimming," and exercises that strengthen the lower trapezius and scapular stability are just a few that often get missed.

I ignore the bottom of my body. It doesn't matter if we are taking a stroll or landing on the ground after making a basketball dunk from the free throw line. The feet and ankles are the first point of force absorption.

I'm not alone with ankle issues. An estimated 25,000 Americans suffer from an ankle sprain each day.[62] Ankle sprains account for almost half of all sports injuries, and up to 20 percent of people who sprain their ankle develop chronic ankle instability.[63] Add in the people who may need a little more mobility because of the impact of modern shoes, and there's more than a few of us who could give some attention to the part of our body that absorbs force first.

We didn't see "perfect ankle" infomercials when we were kids. It's not something that people commonly mention ankles and feet as a problem area with respect to "looks." Yet ankle, foot, and toe function are among the most important things in healthy exercise, risk mitigation, and even performance.[64] [65] [66] [67] Foot and ankle exercises prescribed by a therapist, balancing exercises, and lower leg workouts for the shin and calf are great ways to focus on the bottom of your chain.

I ignore my core. What is the core? This term is everywhere in the fitness industry. Most of us know it's important. But many don't have a complete view.

If abs are the first thing that popped into your head when answering the question above, you're not alone. Marketing has equated abs to the core in product messaging for a long time. Abs are often the most airbrushed and featured part of fitness ads. People in fitness say "squeeze your core" to mean "squeeze your abs."

Perhaps, your answer included the lower back or the trunk. But here's an answer that I'd like you to consider: the core is every muscle that connects to the center of your body (the pelvis) and each is core to your health.

This is the abs *plus* many more muscles such as the inner thighs, quads (thighs), hamstrings, hip rotators, side hips, hip flexors, all of the glutes (including the gluteus medius and minimus), spinal erectors, and key lower back muscles like the quadratus lumborum.

I'm not mentioning these muscles to make this an anatomy book. I'm mentioning them because they are crucial for good health and many of them, when weak or limited, impact the way we absorb force. Many of them, when weak or limited, are also linked to low back pain. It's not standard for people to have a fitness program with strengthening or mobility exercises that give all of these parts dedicated attention.

When I had my paddle boarding incident, I thought my core was strong. I was able to crunch the entire stack of weight on the ab machine at my gym and do planks easily. But I could not stand on the paddle board. I had weakness in the center of my body beyond the abs, and I never focused on balancing exercises or other core exercises that tested the stability of my entire lower chain from the core through the feet.

Our society's confusion about how to define the core holistically and how to measure a strong core means we often do exercises without enough core strength or mobility to help prevent pain or injury.

I ignore muscles that stabilize joints. What if a professional basketball team coach gave 100 percent of his/her attention to a team star and no one else? That would be insane. Every player de-serves attention during practice because their individual roles serve a larger purpose.

Some people exercise like this. The 20 percent of Americans who do strength training exercises often spend most of their time focusing on the Right Swipes and little to none of their time giving dedicated attention to muscles that stabilize the joints. Stability muscles of the foot (a shin muscle called the tibialis anterior), the hip (gluteus medius and piriformis), the spine (psoas), the trunk (erector spinae and side abs), the shoulder blade (serratus anterior) are just a few. Have you seen ads for any of these muscles? Did you hear about them when you were young? It's impossible to care about something if you don't know what it is.

I don't work out my body in all directions. The most popular exercises and machines work the body in four directions: Up, down, backward, and forward. Popular Right Swipe-focused exercises in-clude exercises like squats, dead lifts, bench presses, biceps curls, and shoulder presses. All of them are up and down movements.

Here's the problem: The body moves in *four more directions* that are often ignored or not prioritized: Left, right, right rotation, and left rotation. Those include exercises that move our body laterally or in twists and that are fundamental to joint stability and mobility. Skipping directions is yet another way to create imbalances.

I recently took a popular circuit weight training class with my wife at our gym. It featured 55 minutes of up-down-back-forth movements. There was one minute of bicycle ab crunches (rotation) and one minute of arm side raises (lateral movement). Sadly, this low amount of time allocation to lateral or rotation exercises is common. Some people do zero.

Ads and culture drive priorities to certain areas of the body, which drives a focus on up-and-down or back-and-forth exercises. Lots of key pieces in the chain are ignored with this focus. What that means is that you may be spending a lot of time exercising without optimizing your whole health. It's not a full body workout without lateral or rotational exercises.

Here are a few questions to consider how you spend your time when you aren't doing cardio. Don't worry if you can't answer them immediately. Please just use these questions as a window into how your past has influenced what you do and what you know. It's an opportunity to learn.

- How much of your exercise time is spent rotating or moving laterally?

- Can you name specific foot, ankle, neck, or upper back exercises that you do? Do you do neck mobility exercises (stretches) and calf and shin strengthening or mobility exercises? Do you do balance exercises that gauge lower chain (feet through core) stability? How many exercises or stretches involve putting your arms above your shoulders and rotating them in several directions? Do your feet and shoulders get exercise or stretches in full ranges of motion?

- Do the chest and upper back get equal attention in strength and mobility exercises? Does scapular stability and shoulder mobility and stability get factored into your workouts?

- Do your side abs and low back muscles get as much focus as the front-facing abs? How many of your core exercises are done on your back compared to your belly or sides?

- Does the butt get more focus than the hip flexors (psoas)? Do the side hip muscles and hip rotation get equal attention?

- Do the quads get most of the upper leg focus or do you dedicate some focus to the hamstrings, inner thighs (adductors), and outer hips?

- Have you been guided to check any of these body parts prior to doing more advanced exercises, like pull-ups or lifting heavier weights?

- How often do you do the same types of exercises? (If that number is limited, you are enlisting the same muscles in the same patterns.)

It's common for the (20 percent) minority of people who do strength exercises to skip working out a lot of their muscles. Many of us don't have an exercise plan for the top, middle, and bottom of our body. Weak links may not get fixed. Imbalances may be created when parts are ignored or when unequal attention is given to some parts over others.

Assess your path. If you don't have a head-to-toe strength, mobility, and stability program, are you open to diversifying your fitness routines?

If you have any physical limitations or pain, will you take time to correct them by pausing your current program and seeking medical help or professional guidance?

If you're strong in certain muscles but weak in others and immobile, will you diversify and change?

If not, why? There are exercise programs out there where you can work your entire body at your level.

6

Are Your Cardio Habits as Healthy as You Think?

Cardio is popular. It's what most people do. However, this chapter is meant to answer a question that you may have never asked. Is my cardio routine the best long-term health choice for me or should I take a time out to diversify?

When we look to our fitness past, losing weight, weight loss, trimming, shedding, and slimming are just some of the common phrases used in fitness industry marketing and culture. Often, these words get bundled into a clear message: Doing cardio is how to lose weight. Whether it's done with claims of how many calories you burn or before-and-after pics, the cardio equals weight loss formula is everywhere in fitness.

As a sad sign of the times, I found an ad from a major home equipment brand from 1993 that promised far more than just weight loss from cardio. It said the machine would ease joints, reduce stress, increase energy, improve blood pressure, and boost mental health. That was then. The ad for the same company's updated 2017 model doesn't mention these multiple health outcomes. It sells the machine as being the best for weight loss due to more calories burned. Of course, before and after pictures help make the point visually.

Beyond ads, cardio also is the thing we see the most when we are out on a nice day. We see lots of runners, walkers, and bikers. Tracking how many steps we walk is now part of our culture. We see it everywhere. Running events have increased for decades from 5Ks to half marathons to marathons. Things like the elliptical and home equipment ads have been around as well.

Cardio. Is. Everywhere!

Cardiovascular health is an important health outcome but believing that cardio is the best or the only way to impact health and weight loss should be questioned given how much joint health impacts quality of life.

Consider whether these beliefs apply to you:

Cardio is the most accessible, cheapest, and better than nothing.

When I hear this, and I hear this often from corporate wellness people, it frustrates me. First of all, there are equally accessible and cheaper forms of exercise that provide a more balanced approach to fitness. Things like corrective physical therapy exercises, basic stretches, balancing exercises, basic yoga sun salutations or poses, a simple Pilates side series, or a functional exercise like a bird dog can be learned and done cheaply, anywhere. They can be done in someone's house or a hotel room with no shoes, tracking devices, fancy exercise clothes, or health club memberships required.

As far as the anything-is-better-than-nothing argument, I believe that's like telling someone that by a certain age, they should marry the first person that asks them. Relationships that work are personalized.

That's why I'm frustrated. To me, the anything-is-better-than-nothing argument is a concession to continue to ignore joint health and limit the potential health that people can realize from fitness.

Cardio won't solve or prevent a lot of strength, mobility, or stability problems created by sitting, screen use, and personal history. It can exacerbate them.

Are you willing to take a little time to learn a few simple exercises every month to correct your weak links?

I assume I'm getting a cardio workout.

There's a lot of noise around the word "cardio." People know it's important but they may not know what it is. For example, I saw someone on TV say, "Gardening is great cardio." There are many benefits of gardening, but if you aren't elevating your heart rate enough—which you may or may not be doing while gardening or doing other types of "cardio"—it may not deliver the benefits you think.

I'm not a "maxing out is how to exercise" or a "more is always better" advocate. However, there is a base level of exertion required to gain the benefits of exercise. You need enough resistance with enough reps to fatigue the muscle for proper strength training. You need to elevate your heart rate enough to realize aerobic or aerobic benefits of things like cardio. Become heart rate aware so you can get the most out of your time exercising.

Do you presume you are getting the cardio benefits of exercise or are you measuring your heart rate? There are easy ways to measure if you are, in fact, elevating your heart rate to the right level of intensity: a wearable device or an old-fashioned pulse check.

I don't think about structural health when I focus on cardio.

Cardio can and should be as enjoyable as possible. But excessive cardio, which tends to be the most repetitive form of exercise, can worsen your body's weak links.

The average runner takes 160 to 170 steps per minute.[68] This forces the body to use the same patterns of muscles in the same directions, usually the up-and-down direction, over and over.

Walking, for instance, was bad for my bad ankle and hip. Even the supposedly low-impact elliptical machine stressed my hip. It was too much repetition with compromised parts. Running is a high force, repetitive form of exercise. It's no surprise that running is the cause of many foot, knee, and low back injuries. It's a good idea to research common overuse injuries and how to avoid injury doing your favorite cardio program before you begin exercising.

If you do, you'll find a common theme: Make sure you have strength, stability, and mobility in your lower chain (feet through hips). Also, make sure you have great core strength, good posture, and proper form to avoid injuries and get the most out of your workout.

Have you ever thought of having your walking gait or running form checked? I didn't. Let my pain and medical bills be your incentive. Find out if you have an altered walking or running gait and take the time to correct it. Find out if your lower chain and core are weak in any way.

When I think of "doing cardio," I think of things like running, walking, swimming, cycling, rowing, or doing the elliptical.

Is this statement true for you? These are some ways to elevate the heart rate to realize cardiovascular benefits, but there are other ways. Alternatives like circuit training with weights, kick boxing (or boxing) classes, water aerobics, slam ball classes, or faster yoga like dynamic flow are just a few. There are many ways to elevate the heart rate that don't have the repetition and one-dimensionality of the cultural favorites like running or walking. These alternative workouts can elevate the heart rate while incorporating stability work, dynamic balancing exercises (like kicks or lunges to a single leg balance), strength exercises, and joint mobility training.

Have you tried elevating your heart rate with workouts other than the most common "cardio" exercises?

It's okay to pick up where I left off.

Have you been away from exercise for a while or gained a few pounds? Is your next move to jump in and start running or walking again? Remember that more weight means more absorbed force. And more time off without exercise often means weaker muscles and less mobile joints to absorb those forces in a healthy way.

Physically inactive people can lose as much as 5 percent of their muscle mass each decade after age 30.[69] [70] This is a key reason why strength training is part of fitness guidelines. Time away from exercise is a great reason to focus on structural health as a first fitness priority. Instead of jumping back into a cardio routine, especially if you have a goal of running a 10K or marathon, check first to see what's going on with your body. It's not what most of us do. That's not what ads tell us to do.

Cardio is the best exercise for health and weight loss.

There's a reason why many fitness recommendations have separate strength and aerobic requirements. For example, *The Physical Activity Guidelines for Americans* recommends at least 150 minutes[71] of moderate intensity activity and muscle-strengthening activity at least twice per week for all of the major muscle groups. These guidelines also were endorsed by the American Counsel of Exercise (ACE).[72]

Health benefits for resistance training are different from cardio. Proper resistance training has been linked to improved insulin sensitivity and bone density as well as decreased visceral fat. Resistance training also builds or maintains lean muscle tissue, which we lose as we age.[73] Extra muscle also makes calorie burning easier. It increases your Resting Metabolic Rate (RMR),[74] which relates to the number of calories you burn around the clock when you aren't exercising. This makes it easier to maintain or lose weight.

Eighty percent of people don't do strength training. Do you? Cardio isn't enough to realize the important additional health benefits of resistance training.

Cardio is the easiest form of exercise.

My wife said it best, "Cardio is mindless." That's true. It's really easy to go for a walk or run, sit on a bike, or do the elliptical machine while watching TV. It's also great to put on some music and enjoy the benefits of indoor or outdoor cardio. It's even more mindless if you find a motivational instructor to guide you through a cardio class.

Sometimes we just need a mindless workout to escape. I get it. Please just realize that common cardio is not resistance training, it's not mobility training, and it's not stability training. Popular repetitive cardio doesn't correct a lot of your body's weak links, including those created by excess sitting and screen or device usage.

Repetitive cardio + weak links + bad form + extra mass (body fat or having a larger frame or parts) + years of doing it can turn your fitness path in an unhealthy direction.

Ask yourself:

- Do you spend all or most of your exercise time doing cardio?

- Do you do it without awareness of where your structural health is weak or limited?

- Is it the same type of cardio? If so, do you have a good understanding of your form and function?

- Are you open to diversifying?

- Will you take a time out to shore up your structural health to reduce risks and to get more out of your favorite cardio? If not, why?

7

How Did Others Influence Your Motivation?

We don't get instructions or take classes to figure out which restaurants to visit in our neighborhood, the "good" music to enjoy, which types of movies to like, or which sports teams to cheer for. People close to us show and tell us, free of charge.

People want to share what they care about. It's often a well-intentioned, positive exchange. Nonetheless, it is a process where our relationships with things like food, music, sports, or religion are based on what others around us—including our most trusted sources—value and do.

Our fitness paths are often shaped by the preferences of others too. There's nothing wrong with people sharing the fitness ideas, places, and people that make them happy. In fact, experiences with friends, family, and coaches can be invaluable in developing social skills and bonds with sports or exercises.

However, I learned that it is very important to take an objective look at the power of past or present social experiences.

The first reason is obvious. Negative social fitness experiences may sour someone's relationship with exercise indefinitely.

The second reason is less obvious. Positive social fitness experiences can be so influential that they keep us on a stale or abusive path.

It's true. Positive past social fitness experiences can keep you from pivoting toward health. They did for me.

I was emotional about teaching fitness because I loved the great social engagement. I was emotional about certain workouts because I did them with friends. My father and, sadly, Lance Armstrong made me emotional about cycling. My experiences with friends in school made me emotional about doing exercises that required strong legs or chest. None of this was bad.

But these positive, emotional social experiences drove exercise priorities that resulted in damage to my body. And I kept doing the same things for too long, even after symptoms settled in, because that's what my social experiences taught me to value.

Right now, when you think of fitness, you want certain rewards or outcomes, and those also tend to be based on what you learned from others in your past.

Whatever reward matters most to you, there is something to do—like playing on a team, doing cardio, training for a triathlon, or doing a specific exercise or program—that you likely learned in the past from a trusted source.

In other words, powerful past social experiences are instrumental in shaping the "ratings" of types of exercises that are linked to looks, social or performance outcomes.

Looks ☆ ☆ ☆ ☆ ☆

Performance ☆ ☆ ☆ ☆ ☆

Social ☆ ☆ ☆ ☆ ☆

Measurable Health ☆

Common rewards Linked to social experiences

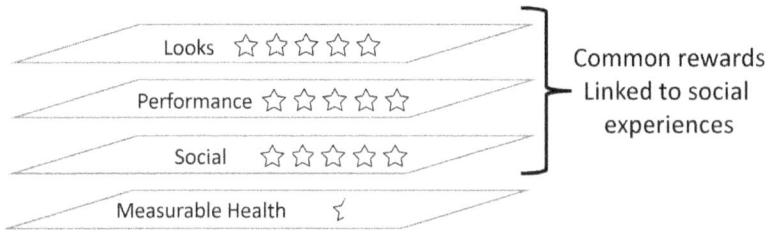

CULTURALLY INFLUENCED RATINGS

Where did you learn to value measurable health outcomes including head-to-toe joint health? How can we rate things like exercises to advance joint health if we lack positive social experiences that showed us what to do and told us why they matter? We can't.

I don't blame the people who shared their methods, workouts, and values with me in my past, but I looked back and saw that the vast majority of my social fitness past did not involve measuring and valuing health outcomes.

That's just a statement of fact.

It's a statement about how much my trusted sources were as much in the dark about structural health as I was because no one taught them.

This chapter is for you to answer this question: how have your social fitness experiences shaped the way you rate measurable health outcomes including joint health versus other fitness rewards?

For many of us, our first exposure to fitness is through recreational games or youth sports. We get exposed to exercise and sports in different ways. I learned to ski and cycle because that's what my dad did. I played youth baseball because that's what was available to kids in my neighborhood.

We also learn about sports and see athletes from the media and advertising. Some of us watch sports games with family and get posters or clothing that feature a favorite athlete or team. We even look up to high school athletes who are invited to elite camps sponsored by major apparel brands. This trend of apparel brands marketing to youth dates back to the 1980s.

We're also exposed to current trends like yoga, obstacle courses, and fitness events with family and friends. The Shamrock Shuffle is an 8K event in Chicago where as many as 30,000 people run and then enjoy food, beer, and music.[75]

The same is true for performance. Even young kids talk about the best exercises to perform or look better. I remember a friend who had posted a note in his bedroom that read, "100 sit-ups a day." He told me he wanted a six pack. We were 12 years old.

How much someone could bench press was a common discussion when I was young. Today, young people are exposed to complicated lifts like a dead lift, squat, or pull-up.

Kids also get the fitness bug from their parents. Many learn to love what their parents do or what their parents encourage.

Then there are social workout experiences, like joining a gym, having friends share their success stories, or hearing about a new fad.

Look back at your social fitness experiences and ask yourself:

- Who influenced the types of sports you played or still play?

- Who influenced the types of exercises you did or still do?

- Do you remember discussions on exercising for certain areas of your body to get a bigger, smaller, or "better" body part?

- What fitness and exercise goals or rewards did you talk about with friends and classmates when you were in school?

- How many of your social experiences related to looks, performance, or social rewards?

- Finally: Did your social influencers specifically talk about valuing health as something to measure and value? How were you taught to measure and track it?

Be careful about believing that losing weight or getting stronger are measurable health outcomes. Of course, strong muscles and weight loss are healthy. However, every time I heard about weight loss or getting stronger when I was young, it related to looks or performance. It was not expressed as a measurable health goal.

I never had any social interactions, whether with friends and family or via the media, that taught me structural health should be a fitness priority to improve performance and reduce injury risk. Things like posture never came up in the context of fitness for me. You, too, may never have been exposed to any other goal of fitness besides those relating to looks, performance, or social outcomes. Or you may have been exposed to fitness rewards that did not prioritize health at all.

It's impossible to prioritize something if we were never taught to value it from cultural and trusted influencers. Even when I was a fitness instructor, I never advised people to measure and prioritize health, like joint health. Culture never taught my influencers to prioritize it.

Please do not discount the power of social experiences over many years, dating back to your youth, in influencing your motivation where health is not the highest priority.

It's not just the major social influences, however. The social rewards of fitness can also be tiny but incredibly powerful. In his book, *The Power of Habit*, author Charles Duhigg uses a story about a survey done for the YMCA to highlight how small social interactions influence our motivations.

"While a facility's (gym) attractiveness and the availability of workout machines might have caused people to join in the first place…retention, the data said, was driven by emotional factors such as whether employees know members' names or said hello when they walked in," he writes. "People…often go to the gym looking for a human connection, not a treadmill."

Why is this a big deal? I want you to have positive social fitness experiences. I hope you love the people and the places where you exercise. But I want you to be aware that even little social rewards like these can stop you from diversifying your fitness routine if your health demands it.

The reality is that sometimes the healthiest program may require a shift and you can find new positive social experiences if you take the time to try. Be open to how powerful social experiences can get in the way of needed change. Such experiences may date back to your youth where your influencers weren't taught how to guide you to measure and correct your weak links as a first priority.

Ask yourself:

- How powerful are the past or present social rewards in your fitness world? How much did positive fitness experiences influence your current motivation? What do they drive you to do?

- Are you currently emotionally anchored to doing a specific workout at a specific place or exercising in the same way with the same people?

- Do your emotional goals prevent you from trying new things, places, and people that can improve the trajectory of your health? If yes, why?

8

Performance or Health—
What Matters More?

Most of us have heard about finding "The One" in the context of a romantic relationship. Some people have found their "One" in fitness—a favorite type of exercise or sport that they love and do the most. It makes them feel good. It's the thing above all other fitness or sports-related activities that they associate with success and pursuing their dream.

People talk about "dream" bodies and "dream" achievements in fitness and sport cultures. It's common for people to get excited and emotional about these Better, Bigger, Faster, Stronger, or (enduring) Longer performance or achievement goals—BBFSL goals, as I call them.

When I looked back, I realized that a lot of my fitness happiness had to do with being able to achieve outcomes that I could show off to others. Showy goals are the most advertised goals. Showy goals are dream goals, and they can keep people on stale or abusive paths by overriding logic and a focus on health.

This chapter is meant for you to answer these questions: Are your dreamy, BBFSL goals more important than your long-term health? Is pursuing those goals tuning your health negatively in any way, including your structural health? Finally, when did you first develop these BBFSL goals?

The word "dream" appears all over fitness ads and conversations, along with dreamy synonyms like "epic," "eternal," "greatness," and "legendary."

We also hear the word "hero" used to describe the best performers and winners. And how awesome is it to become an "Un?" Unstoppable. Unbreakable. Unforgettable. Unbelievable. Words like "valor" and "glory" also are staples of fitness and sport BBFSL marketing, particularly in fitness apparel ads for major brands.

Being better is another constant fitness theme. Victory. Winning. Champion. They are all showy proof of being better. We've talked about winning and being better since we followed sports teams and played games as kids. And we're seeing more and more intense challenges like triathlons, power-lifting-based workouts, and even more complex obstacle courses.

Fighting metaphors are common in marketing and sports conversations. You've seen competitive words like combat, protect, vengeance, revenge, and dominate show up regularly in ads and sports coverage on TV. We also talk about school and team rivalries which further cement emotional bonds to sports.

The concept of better also relates to self-improvement and personal bests. Words like "pride," "shine," and "commitment" are esteem-building ingredients in fitness advertising. The word "impossible" pops up often. What better way to build esteem than to do the impossible?

All of these experiences underscore our emotional connection to the aesthetic, performance, and social rewards of fitness. These marketed associations provide powerful emotional reinforcement to ratings developed through social experiences. You may have learned to get emotional about your favorite sport or exercise from a friend, family member, or coach. Marketing then takes this already highly rated association and elevates its value to you.

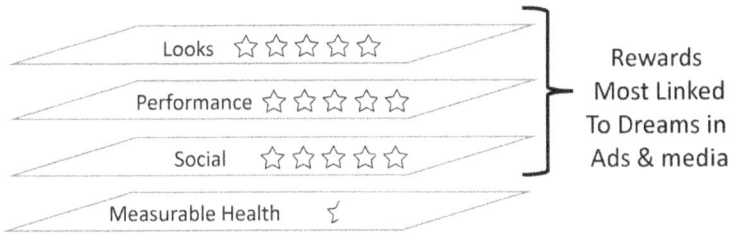

These words then get linked to other marketed concepts like harder, extreme, and badass—things revered by many in fitness.

They also get linked to people, like sports champions and fitness celebrities, who have become "the one" who embodies the ultimate achievement because they've won the ultimate trophy, medal, or championship. Seeing others realize dreamy goals that we want can get us emotional about a sport or goal. That's why top performers are paid top endorsement contracts.

The rewards for being better are mighty. It could be money (especially if you're a successful professional athlete), fame, or attention from peers.

That's just a small sample of common things we've seen and heard from the media, marketing, and ads to jog your memory.

Here are some things to consider:

- What are your BBFSL fitness or sports goals?

- How emotionally tied are you to these goals? What about them seems aspirational to you?

- Before you pursued these goals, did you consider having your structural health assessed?

BBFSL goals and their emotional value can override your desire or willingness to make any changes for the sake of your health. I know. That was me and many like me who want to keep doing the thing that they are good at or the thing that is most coveted culturally.

For example, I also could lift multiple times my body weight on the leg press machine. Though I wouldn't win any strength competitions, I could lift more than most people in the gym. However, I struggled squatting half of my body weight. In fact, I squatted far less weight than many people. What accounted for the difference? The leg press machine stabilizes the body's up-and-down movement. But a free-weight, barbell squat makes the body, particularly the lower chain, stabilize the up-and-down movement. I didn't have lower chain stability so I didn't do squats. The leg press machine made me feel good. I was "good" at it. Again, I focused on the exercise that made me feel good for years instead of figuring out why I couldn't squat.

In my small fitness circle, I know many other people who put BBFSL goals over health. In fact, I met a therapist who hurt her body running marathons and another therapist who loved dead lifts and ignored her lower back weakness from a car accident. She reinjured herself doing dead lifts. I have a friend who is an accomplished triathlete who won't stop running, even after a diagnosis of torn knee ligaments. Others I know can link their knee and foot issues to running and won't stop.

People everywhere are tuning joint health in the wrong direction in the name of BBFSL goals. I valued what my fitness past told me to value: Better, Bigger, Faster, Stronger, and Longer.

Ask yourself:

- Are you doing the same thing?

- Do you favor exercises that showcase your strengths versus learning new things?

- Are you teaching your kids to do the same?

Kids can learn a lot of good life skills through competitive sports. Teamwork, accountability, and communication are just a few. But it's also important to talk to kids about head-to-toe structural health because sports injuries are all too common.

In fact, nearly half of all sports injuries among middle and high school students are due to muscle overuse or repeating a movement over and over. This dovetails with a trend in youth sports for specialization—playing the same sport more versus changing sports over the course of the year.

As a 2018 article on AARP.org noted, "[If] a child is spending more than eight months annually in one sport, he or she is nearly three times more likely to experience an overuse injury in their hip or knee."[76]

But it's not just overuse that can cause injuries. They can also happen when weak links aren't assessed and corrected before engaging in high force sports activities. If there are no structural health assessments of kids before they participate in sports, how would they or their parents know?

There are other things that aren't part of common knowledge or consideration. For example, females tear the anterior cruciate ligaments (ACL) in the knee 3.5 times more than males in basketball and 2.8 times more than males in soccer.[77] Clearly, the sheer physics of landing on a leg is different for males compared to females. Where is the process to measure young females and males and account for their function, form, and physics?

Also, there is more than enough information that shows the risk of injury is higher when you have a weak core.[78] But who guides young people to define and measure the core before sending their bodies in motion?

There certainly is a lot of how-to-play-the-game coaching in youth sports but what about the how-to-prepare-the-body-to-play-the-game coaching? Did you get it in your youth? Do your kids?

This is important because people like me who develop dreamy BBFSL motivations when we are young get older, remaining unaware of our weak links. We continue with our preference for higher force exercises, harder cardio, or Right Swipe BBFSL training programs because that's what we learned to value when we were young. Sports and competitive passion from our youth evolves into a drive for marathons and triathlons. Same emotional performance rewards, different way to get them.

Other than kids, there are people who use BBFSL achievement as a proxy for youth. In fact, our culture glorifies the ability to continue to do hard workouts as we age. If this is you, I hope that you are factoring in your structural health and answering the questions in these chapters seriously. Your tuning should dictate what goals you should pursue if health is what you truly care about.

I found out retroactively, for me and many people I know, that feeling good about dreamy BBFSL goals in our twenties, thirties, forties, and fifties can have a negative impact on the quality of the final chapters of our lives. We've bought into the notion that more is always better.

The concept of doing more is often valued in fitness: Longer workouts. More weight. More distance. More (and extreme) flexibility in yoga poses. However, more doesn't always translate to better health. In fact, there are studies that show how intense endurance training is bad for health.[79] At some point, more distance can translate into negative tuning not just for the joints but for the heart.[80] [81] There are concerns that overdoing yoga and forcing prescribed poses, instead of doing modifications, is causing hip issues in yoga instructors.[82]

People can get injured when they push beyond their level with the belief that more is always better.

Do you recall experiences where you learned that more equaled better for fitness or sports? Do you believe more is better for long-term health? If so, what measurable short- or long-term method are you using to quantify how more is better from a health perspective?

You also may believe that certain exercises like physical therapy exercises, tai chi, yoga, or Pilates are not "real" or of lesser value than the BBFSL workouts. If that's the case, please let go of this unfortunate belief. I recommended Pilates to a woman in her thirties who was a former competitive athlete. She told me that she had knee pain and couldn't do her high intensity exercises anymore. She laughed off my suggestion of Pilates, saying it wasn't a "real" exercise. But basic exercises are neither real, right, wrong, good, or bad. They are indicators of your ability to control and stabilize your body. Athletes like NBA player Lebron James embrace yoga.[83] Pilates, too, is getting more acceptance in baseball because of how beneficial it is for full body performance.[84]

If you believe that these exercises like Pilates, barre, or yoga are inferior for any reason or if you believe that they are just stretching exercises, I challenge you to stop labeling exercises and start using exercises as indicators of your body's health.

Ask yourself:

- Will you change if your BBFSL goals are not headed toward health or if you are experiencing pain?

- Will you change if you know that your BBFSL goals are the source of a health issue?

- If you have a BBFSL or sport preference, will you take a time out to shore up your structural health and form as a first priority? If not, why?

9

Did Fitness Get Painful Physically or Emotionally?

P ain is a fitness topic that we don't talk about enough. I'm not talking just about injury. This chapter is about two extreme ends of fitness, where you or someone you know has:

- Bought into the "no pain, no gain" mantra and keeps doing exercises that cause physical pain.

- Had emotionally painful fitness experiences that made them feel excluded from fitness, even to the point where they "hate" exercise.

It's one thing to let social or BBFSL experiences steer your fitness journey to a point of pain or injury. It's another to ignore it or value pain as a badge of courage and keep going. Nothing says fitness is not about health more than celebrating and continuing fitness habits that cause pain or injury.

If you look at as many fitness ads as I have, you'll clearly see that pain is advertised as a virtue. Some fitness ads that I've seen proudly use the concept of pain in ways that are paraphrased as follows:

- Linking pain with pride.

- Positively describing pain as fuel to drive people ahead.

- Pushing through pain and then pushing more.

- Showcasing pain as a reward.

- Advocating that hurting is part of "working."

- Ignoring tears in favor of results.

- Calling pain an excuse to not keep pursuing BBFSL goals.

Some fitness enthusiasts have even adopted the US Marine mantra of "Pain is weakness leaving the body" on their social media posts. To be clear, our valiant service members need to train their minds to function while experiencing pain and injury. Their life or the life of someone in their unit may be on the line.

But let's be honest. There's a difference between taking hostile enemy fire in a foreign land and training for a half marathon because you're turning 40.

It's also common to hear fans and the sports media celebrate athletes playing through pain. These performances are hyped as being courageous, even though this is the job of athletes who make millions of dollars. That messaging can be a harmful influence on ordinary women and men, including those without elite athlete access to medical care and trainers.

There's nothing wrong with working hard. In fact, as I mentioned earlier, the benefits of exercise often happen when we get out of our comfort zone, like when we increase our heart rate doing cardio or work to fatigue while lifting weights.

While fatigue can be healthy, the problem is that people generally aren't taught the difference between fatigue and pain.[85] [86] [87] Please learn the difference. For example, fatigue in the quads during a set of squats can be good. The muscle is doing work. Pain in the knees or back during a squat means you should stop squatting.

Pain. Should. Not. Be. Ignored. It's a red flag to change your exercise program. But many people head the call from fitness ads and culture to not let pain get in the way of more-is-better looks or performance goals.

An article on CNN.com titled, "Yes you can run a half marathon after knee and back injuries"[88] features the story of a 47-year-old doctor who said she had a list of prior injuries that "reads like a medieval saga." She mentions numerous back and knee injuries that result in three surgeries and dozens of injections. Plus, she admits to having an unstable knee. Still, she writes that she "always dreamed of running a half marathon." There is proof that dreamy goals are alive and well in fitness culture!

On she ran, but she experienced knee inflammation and then terrible back pain. Off she went to the chiropractor, who recommended a running coach to help correct poor form. (Poor form, I might add, that she never had assessed or corrected prior to starting.)

She concludes that she enjoyed celebrating with her family. Also, that people should receive training and medical support to avoid injury. But she didn't avoid an injury! She already had injuries. Pursuing her dreamy fitness goal created a need to see a chiropractor, just like pursuing performance fitness goals has driven me and so many others to drive up the cost of health care. Still, we celebrate the achievement and ignore that fitness, which is proclaimed to be healthy, is a source of injury to our bodies with to-be-determined, long-term consequences.

I hate to single out this doctor because I don't want to deflect from taking ownership of my own fitness failure. But it's an example that shows how we consider health relative to socially constructed rewards.

Do you or do you know someone who:

- Has severe pain or impaired performance because of an issue?

- Knows that their fitness choices are the root of a clinical issue with symptoms like swelling?

- Feels the impact of exercise in the form of aches or pains long after they are done exercising?

If the answer is yes, will you or the person you know:

- Stop for a while, or indefinitely, depending the condition's severity? I had to walk away from my favorite exercises.

- Get assessed and see if buttressing your structural health or improving form can lessen or eliminate the symptoms?

- If not, why?

Seriously, if you know that your favorite sport or exercise hurts your body or if you know it's stressful on an already compromised body part, why do you keep doing it? What's really in it for you?

I ignored pain for 10 years. Gravity won. It always does. I allowed people and companies, who won't be around to help me when my health ebbs in my senior years, influence what I cared about in the short term.

Just as fitness can feel great for an "in crowd" who have had success, there are others who feel emotional pain because fitness or sports-related experiences made them feel excluded or frustrated.

People can feel left out of fitness if they aren't able to do something. Even things like walking 10,000 steps can make people feel like part of the "out crowd" if walking hurts. This was my experience. I talked to a business colleague who told me that he also stopped walking because he felt pain in his knee and hip.

It can be more than a little discouraging to try to do something like walking and then have to stop because it hurts. It made me feel old. Welcome to the unspoken reality of fitness culture and marketing, which talks a lot about success. It doesn't talk about why people leave fitness and don't come back.

It's easy for fitness pros to make statements like "no excuses." But there's more to it. As much as people get positively emotional about fitness with good experiences, the opposite can be true.

An August 2018 *New York Times* article highlighted a study that showed how "memories of physical education classes are both common and consequential."[89] The study was based on an online questionnaire that included an opportunity to provide the "single best or worst memory from a PE class and write about it in as much detail as they chose."

The results showed that "people who had not enjoyed gym class as children tended to report that they did not expect to exercise now and did not plan to exercise in the coming days. People who had found pleasure in gym class, on the other hand, were more likely to report that they expected exercise to be enjoyable and that they were active on weekends."

I would bet that the same holds true for people who had positive or negative experiences in youth sports. This is another example of what a powerful influence the experiences of our youth can exert on our later life.

Others may remember the humiliating process of picking teams in gym class, where some kids were always picked last. Others got hit in the head with a dodge ball or were teased for any number of reasons, including their weight or ability. It was even worse if an authority figure like a coach or gym teacher singled a kid out. These painful experiences get linked to fitness for life![90]

Were sports and games your first introduction to fitness? How did they influence you?

Did you have gym classes that were largely focused on games, sports, learning sports skills, or running a certain distance in a certain time? Were those experiences positive or negative? Or did you learn the fundamentals of full-body exercise, including stability and mobility work? Were those experiences positive or negative?

Even experiences like showing up to a fitness class that's not taught at your level can be frustrating. Having entry-level classes, even for complicated things like kettlebells, is not a standard at all gyms. People can be made to feel like they can't keep up because an advanced class or program doesn't adapt to their level. Is it really someone's fault if they feel like they don't know how to exercise when there's no one to teach them fundamentals?

Emotionally hurtful or frustrating experiences like these can grow to a point where people say, "I hate exercise." I never thought about "hating exercising" until researching and writing this book. My wife hated exercise for years. She remembers getting hit in the face with a volleyball during gym classes and feeling embarrassed.

Do you feel like your fitness past is filled with experiences where people didn't teach you at your level or where you felt excluded or dispirited for any reason, including how you looked?

If so, you may have been made to feel:

- Exercise is not for me.

- I hate exercise.

- I don't know how to exercise.

- Exercise hurts.

- I don't fit in.

- I try but fail at exercise.

If any of this holds true for you, divorcing your fitness past is a must. You can't succeed in fitness if your path doesn't first involve assessing and coming to terms with your influences.

10

Have Ads Blocked Your Long-Term Health Goals?

Relationships can fail when people expect too much too soon. In fitness, the industry's marketing and culture drives us to fast results. They know we want them so they tell us it's possible.

This final chapter about your fitness past is to answer serious questions about your fitness goals and expectations: Are they short-sighted? And are you willing to take a step back to build a long-term plan that may require changes, big or small, depending on where you are?

The fitness industry markets time to their financial advantage. This is typically the magazine, infomercial, and product purveyors like fitness magazines, machines, and programs.

We have been inundated with these messages for decades on TV, in gyms, and in line at grocery stores and airports.

The industry knows great marketing grabs your attention by communicating a payoff that you care about and how to get it... fast.

The more quickly you think you can get the reward, the more inclined you are to want it. Results are the payoff, and the ways to get it include workouts and equipment.

Then marketers use time frames like 3, 6, 30, 60, or 90 days, which makes the payoff seem within reach. Coupled with a before and after picture, the pitch is even more powerful and our wallet comes out.

Words like fast, quick, and now are everywhere in fitness marketing. Sometimes these claims are linked to fitness celebrities, Hollywood celebrities, and top athletes in ads, on social media, or on magazine covers.

We hear about fast results more from advertising than from trusted people in our lives, but we also hear people talk about losing weight by the date of a specific event like a wedding. It may seem subtle but setting timed fitness or weight loss goals is just another way culture teaches us to put fitness on a clock. A clock that often runs for less than 90 days—a time frame that is less than realistic or healthy.

Have you ever set a long-term health goal with a measurable outcome? Something specific to health other than weight loss (which is often a looks-related goal), like improved checkup scores or joint health?

Here's the problem with short-term expectation fitness. Imagine going to a couple's therapist who never met you or your partner and said your relationship would be fixed in 30 days. As crazy as it sounds, that's how many of us set fitness expectations.

The most damaging cultural impact from the promise of "fast results" is that our expectations for things to come quickly become unhealthy.

Some people may have to build several healthy eating habits that may take a long time. Others may need to address how stress, mental health, or sleep issues impact their lives. Some people start with structural health issues, which may take a lot of time to correct. Without considering what is both healthy and realistically possible, people set themselves up for some combination of failure, frustration, dejection, or injury.

Do you see the problem? Not only do people want something fast that's often a distant goal but what they want is often emotional. These emotional expectations don't take into account limiting personal factors.

I have a friend in his fifties who hadn't exercised in years. He bought an intense, 60-day, at-home DVD program. He did two days and was in pain for four more. He was so turned off that he stopped. I know others who have been injured taking a hard class for which they didn't have to qualify.

There's another potential problem with fast results: Losing weight too quickly also is unhealthy. Some people change their metabolism and when they do, they're more likely to put weight back on. Others go on extreme, all-or-nothing diets like zero sugars or "no cheat days" and don't build sustainable habits.

I've seen and heard so many people make today's workouts about maximizing short-term looks or performance results. I've met lifters who worry they'll get smaller if they take a week or day off. People have told me to give them a harder workout before the weekend or prior to a holiday in preparation for the food and drinks to come.

It's generally not part of our fitness culture to care about assessing and advancing health gradually from an individual starting point. It's also not common to celebrate incremental gains.

Please consider and be open to how your past experiences have
not guided you to value an incremental learning process or taught
you how to build a long-term approach. Constant exposure to fast
results claims in fitness marketing may play a bigger role in your
fitness expectations than you think. The good news is that there is
time to change.

SUMMARY

Are You on a Healthy Fitness Path?

Y ou may not be maximizing short- or long-term health outcomes when one or more of these statements applies to you:

- You are unaware of where you are weak, unstable, mobility-limited, or imbalanced in your body.

- You are not actively working on correcting these weak links, if you are aware of them. Instead, you keep doing exercises where you are already strong.

- You've been so dispirited by the fitness industry that you've given up the pursuit of fitness.

- You no longer care about looks or performance rewards, but you've never been guided to measure or care about health rewards.

- You do an exercise regularly without having your form professionally checked, even while walking.

- You don't have a long-term health focus.

- You believe exercise is a huge part of a weight loss solution, even if you've unsuccessfully tried to rely on exercise to maintain a desired weight.

- One type of cardio is your predominant or exclusive exercise focus.

- Non-cardio exercises focus on Right Swipe parts while ignoring stability or range (mobility).

- You do the same cardio or strength exercises every week and month, repeatedly working the same patterns of muscles in the same ranges of motion. Nothing says your relationship is stale more than a lack of diversity and lack of exploring new types of exercises that can test and advance your structural health.

- Fitness regimens have injured you but you haven't changed and may even take pride in the pain.

- You presume your program is healthy without measuring it, particularly when it comes to your head-to-toe joint health.

- You are so emotionally tied to your program that you won't take a time out or pivot to new exercises.

In the previous chapters, I've shared how beliefs and motivation can fuel habits that can keep you on an unhealthy fitness path. I'd like to share one more: The belief that you don't need to change.

Sadly, I believed this for decades, even when I needed a radical change in my priorities and program.

I now believe:

- I was caught up in a culture that hasn't developed a standard way to measure and prioritize health.

- I was once illogical and emotionally biased when it came to fitness, both as a young man and as an instructor.

If, like me, you're finally open to change, then it's time for a reboot!

PART 3

Things to Learn and Accept
Before Moving On

If you're open to changing a lifetime of fitness habits in the name of health, then it's time to move on.

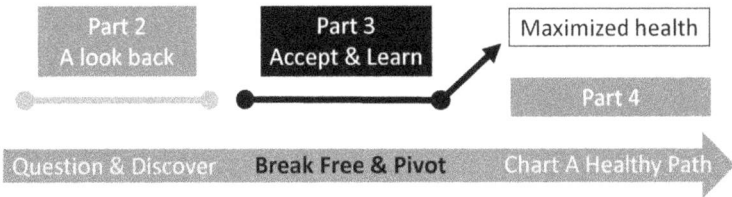

However, there are some things that need to happen after a "breakup" with old habits. We need to accept where we are, watch out for traps that keep us in the past, and learn some basics about what it takes to be on a new, healthier path.

The next three quick chapters are about:

- Accepting that fitness advertising has deliberately tied you emotionally to rewards other than health (Chapter 11).

- Understanding and recognizing biases that can keep you rationalizing you path (Chapter 12).

- Learning the fundamentals of replacing bad habits and how to build new ones in preparation for Part 4 (Chapter 13).

11

Ads Did Not Get Us Emotional About Health

Whatever your opinion about advertising, the reality is that marketing is everywhere because it works. Companies wouldn't spend $600 billion dollars in 2018[91] if it didn't.

Hopefully, you paused a little in Part 2 to reflect on a cultural reality: it's not a coincidence that what is advertised influences our knowledge, motivation, habits, and priorities.

Before moving on, it's important to understand and accept some important facts about marketing:

1. The way we associate concepts in our memory influences our beliefs, reactions, and behaviors.

2. Advertisers focus on building specific associations.

3. The fitness industry, including the sports media, purposely builds emotional and aspirational associations with their brands, workouts, teams, and products—mostly linked to the rewards of looks, performance, or social outcomes.

4. Fitness marketing and advertising doesn't have to directly
    impact you to influence you. It can influence you subtly,
    gradually, and indirectly.

This chapter is a quick overview of how and why fitness advertising influences the relative and lower rating of health compared to
the most advertised fitness rewards.

Let's start with an important fact about memory. Memory isn't
like a room of fixed, compartmentalized records. Researchers have
shown that memory is associative, where one thing gets linked to
other things which then gets linked, or associated, to other things.[92]
Your favorite music artist isn't filed in an isolated music memory
folder. It's linked to people, places, sights, sounds, (possibly smells),
and feelings where you experienced the music. These associations—
the way we link concepts—highly influence our beliefs, feelings, and
motivation.

I came across an interesting behavioral study to illustrate how
powerful this is.[93] In English, all nouns have one article: *The*. For
example, we say *the* key or *the* bridge. Some languages, like Spanish
and German, have what are called masculine and feminine nouns,
each of which has a different article, like "*el*" and "*la*" in Spanish.
Social scientists asked people in these cultures to give three adjec-
tives to describe a given noun. They wanted to determine if learning
words as being masculine or feminine impacted cultural associations.
It did. Take a look at the chart below to see the link between what
we learn in culture and how our minds associate concepts.

Article with Word	Language/ (Masculine or Feminine)	Adjectives associated with the word
The Key (der schüssel)	German/masculine	Hard, heavy, jagged, metal and useful
The Key (la llave)	Spanish/feminine	Golden, intricate, little, lovely and tiny
The Bridge (die brucke)	German/feminine	Beautiful, elegant, fragile, pretty and slender
The Bridge (el puente)	Spanish/masculine	Big, dangerous, strong, sturdy and towering

You can see that simply labeling these nouns as masculine or feminine, concepts with built-in mental links to other associated concepts learned in culture, changes the way people think of things.

This is what advertising does: it links words, images, and concepts that already have built-in, favorable associations in our mind to the promoted brand, product, idea, politician, or whatever.

Advertisers want to tap into our associative memory and build connections to existing, powerful concepts.

Advertising also influences our relative, emotional ranking of concepts or things. I'd like to show you how by using Maslow's hierarchy of needs as a guide. Abraham Maslow, an American psychologist, created this motivation framework to show how humans, though different, share a framework of needs that we live to satisfy.

Transcendence	Sharing our potential with others
Self Actualization	Realizing our **human potential**
Aesthetics	Presentation of our **looks**, house, garden
Cognitive	Learning, Discovering, Exploring
Esteem	**Status, awards, recognition, winning**
Love & Belonging	**Clubs, teams**, relationships, family
Safety	**Health**, shelter, physical safety
Physiological	Water, food, sleep

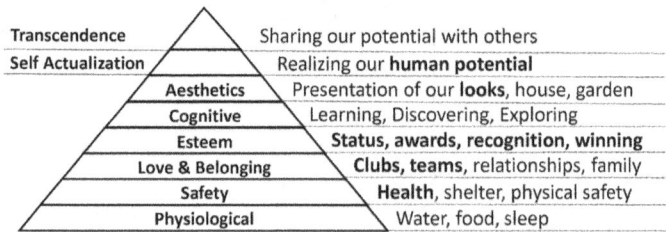

MASLOW'S HIERARCHY OF NEEDS

It works like this: Humans have needs. We are motivated to fulfill those needs. Our survival needs at the base of the pyramid have to be sufficiently fulfilled for us to get our higher-level emotional and social needs met.

For example, we would not care about getting a date for Saturday night if we were dehydrated and starving. Dehydration and starvation are examples of major physiological deficiencies that constitute basic, lower level needs.

Health does not live at the top of the pyramid. It lives at the bottom at the safety level. In fitness, if we are seriously injured, we have no choice but to start here.

But what happens when we are not seriously lacking in our most basic safety and physiological needs? We tend to spend a lot of time, energy, and money focused on fulfilling our higher-level needs, starting with our love and belonging and our esteem needs.

Our attention jumps right past the bottom two survival levels, where health lives, when things at the base of the pyramid are "good enough." Why? We are emotional. And many of our emotional needs require interaction with other people to become fulfilled.

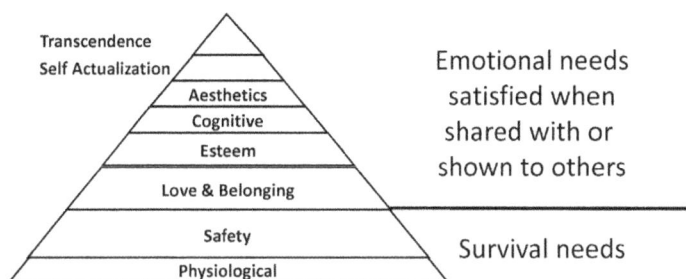

Think about our consumer culture. We purchase luxury items to enhance our esteem or spend money socializing with friends, even if we can't afford them. In other words, we jeopardize our personal safety—including our economic stability—for the sake of fulfilling short-term higher, social, and esteem needs. We do the same when we buy clothes or beauty products for aesthetic need fulfillment.

This is critical to understanding how marketing influences fitness choices and priorities. If our health is "good enough," then we want to climb the ladder for emotional fulfilment. It's not surprising that fitness marketing and ads target upper levels of the pyramid, skipping or deprioritizing health.

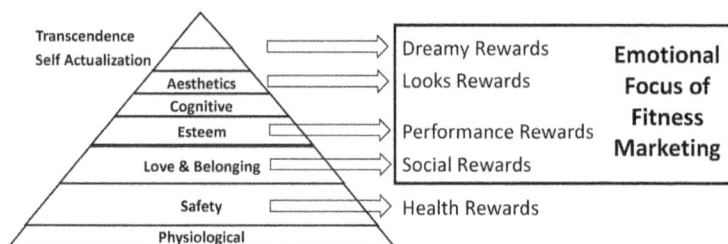

Why do they do this? When ads generate an emotional response, they sell more products and build more allegiance to brands.[94] [95] You've heard that sex sells. Well, emotions sell. A 2016 Nielsen report found that ads with the best emotional response generate a 23% lift in sales.[96] It works on all of us but consider the power of targeting emotions when talking about looks and fitness performance rewards to impressionable young people. Young people who are less likely to have health issues and who haven't had the joy of experiencing gravity for decades. Since you were young, ads and culture built emotional associations to fitness high up the pyramid.

All of the advertising words and examples I used in Part 2 are ways to target emotions from the social (love and belonging) level up through the dreamy, aspirational top of Maslow's pyramid.

Health, which has lower emotional value to people who don't have health issues, is often left out of ads. Or it's a side show to the featured rewards higher in the pyramid. Putting the word health in a fitness ad or magazine cover next to a hot body or image that depicts extreme performance is like giving a kid socks for Christmas with a great toy or device. Sure, it's there. But it's not fun or memorable.

The combination of brands wanting to build aspirational associations, the power of selling emotions, the huge impact of communicating the rewards visually, and the fact that targeting younger people is a proven method to maximize profits are key reasons why many of us are emotional about everything other than health on our fitness path.

The influence of fitness marketing on us doesn't happen overnight. It takes time and money to bring awareness to a point where culture values new things and changes behavior.

You may not lift weights or want muscles because you saw an ad. However, there's a long trail back to Arnold Schwarzenegger's *Pumping Iron* movie in 1977, all of the muscle magazines, all of the muscular Hollywood leading men in the 80s, and all of the exposure to lifting in gyms over the years. There were also lots and lots of ads featuring muscles over decades.

Running also started small. The sport has military roots but became popular partly due to the landmark 1968 book *Aerobics* by Ken Cooper that helped launch the running craze. Since then, there have been tons of running and running apparel ads along with friends and family who praise the value of running. So let's say someone tries it. Then they get social, esteem, and physical rewards. Then ads come along and link the concepts of pride, perseverance, eternal, excel, strong, endure, better, glory, and greatness to running. The models in the ads are lean so running also gets weight loss associations. Now running has more linked associations. Associations that are emotional.

Ads don't make us run or make us pick our favorite exercises or sport. The ads tap into powerful associations in our memory, which then make our fitness choices more meaningful in our life.

Most important, and the reason for this chapter, these associations make our preferred exercises or sports harder to walk away from if we need a time out or pivot for health.

What I want you to realize is that marketing and the media to some degree influenced your emotional associations with fitness—directly, indirectly, or both. And the more you are aware of that, the easier it will be to break bad habits and reclaim your health.

It took over 50 years of public messages, and a ban of cigarette ads on TV and radio in 1969, to get the percentage of adults who smoke in America from 42.4 percent in 1965 to 14 percent in 2017.[97] As I mentioned earlier, there have been zero widespread, national campaigns guiding people to consider or factor long-term joint health in relation to exercise.

So start accepting that ads influenced your fitness preferences and become your own health advocate.

12

Fitness Biases Are Real and Limit Health

What if we went to a high-end dating or matchmaking service to find our true love? The process would work like this: we sign up for the service and state our list of preferred qualities in our desired match.

The service then runs an algorithm that has been programmed in the past to automatically predict the "best" match for us. The "best" option predicted by the algorithm:

- Needs to be a person that was already programmed in the system as a viable option.

- And uses a rating system based on what presumably worked for other people.

This makes the system biased to both the limited scope of the people in the database and its automatic rating system that doesn't really know us. Well, the brain often works like a similarly biased "matchmaker" for fitness. It doesn't always choose the best or healthiest option. Instead, the brain often prefers the familiar or easy options.

This quick chapter is about accepting the possibility that there are irrational biases that keep you on the same path, particularly if your fitness rewards are emotional. The brain will unthinkingly repeat behaviors in autopilot mode unless you consciously recognize and accept your biases. I know they are real because I know I was biased too. I saw it all around fitness.

It's important to realize that the brain is highly influenced by repetition, which makes things more memorable. But memory, as discussed in the last chapter, isn't just about knowing or recalling things, it's associative.

The brain uses these associations to predict information, like the GPS-enabled directions app on your phone takes predictive short-cuts. If you type the letters H and O in your mapping app, it will not only predict "home" as what you want but it fills in the best way to get there. This "best way" has been learned from past experiences when your phone calculated the time and best route to get home.

That's how the brain works: It uses a lot of our calories (20 percent of our total caloric intake) and wants to use that energy as efficiently as possible.[98] As a result, we evolved an autopilot brain function mode to handle known and familiar routines to get known rewards, like how to get home. This mode saves us energy and helps us survive. It's a nifty prediction engine to tell us the easiest way to fulfill our needs—picking the highest rated reward and routine to get that reward if multiple options are available.

Our autopilot heavily relies on past experiences where we pro-grammed our associations among people, places, and things. We then linked these associated concepts to specific rewards and routines to get them.

Let me share an experiment to highlight how this works. Neuroscientist Ann Graybiel and her lab at the Massachusetts Institute of Technology (MIT) led a neurological study of habits on rats[99] [100] that showed how the brain learns to operate in autopilot mode with repetition. They hooked up the rats' brains to a machine that measured neural activity and put the rat at the start of a simple T-shaped maze (see diagram) with a piece of chocolate in the same place for all trials. Then they opened a gate that separated the rat from the maze.

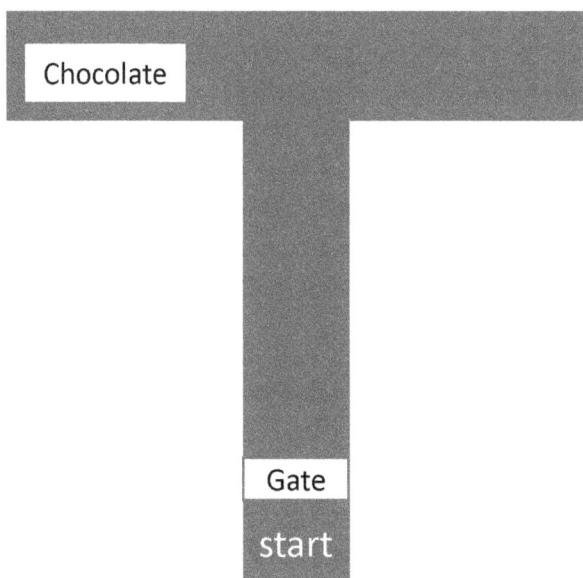

The first few times, the rat had lots of neural activity during three phases: When the gate opened, during the routine trip through the T, and then when it found the chocolate. However, after going through the maze repetitively, there was only a spike in neural activity in two parts: When the rat heard the gate and when it got to the chocolate. Neural activity was otherwise "quiet" while the rat went through the maze because it learned the routine of getting through the maze in autopilot mode.

That's how I'm defining autopilot mode: A process where a triggering event—some combination of associated concepts like people, places, or things like sounds or emotions—causes our brain to automatically predict associated rewards and things to do to get them after enough repetition.

How you gauge the best exercises is likely an autopilot response "programmed" in your memory over years, when measurable health outcomes may not have been getting a lot of thought or consideration. Chocolate isn't the reward for fitness. Instead, looks, performance, and social rewards lie at the end of our associative fitness memory maze. These outcomes were programmed with repetitive exposure in your past, including powerful emotional associations learned through social experiences and with great ads. This puts health outcomes and the routines to get them at a big neural disadvantage.

Right now, the things you value most from fitness and what to do to get there are programmed like superhighways in your neural mind map. The things to do for health, like prioritizing physical therapy or learning something new like yoga or Pilates, are likely programmed as less important side streets, alleys, or even hiking paths.

I can't tell you how important it is to recognize that a shift in exercise motivation and goals is hard. It's hard because it's not natural for many of us to care about exercising for health as a first priority. Our past didn't program our associative memory to care. Taking those first two Pilates classes or doing those therapy exercises for the first few weeks won't feel as rewarding as other known-and-valued workouts or sports. They will only feel rewarding after you do them enough to feel and value measurable health results.

If you don't put in the time to learn new things to improve health, not only will you not get the health rewards, you may rationalize what you do. The reason is that our autopilot mode is error-pronged and full of cognitive biases that have been studied and validated by experts for decades.

Confirmation bias, for instance, is a well-known cognitive bias. It's a tendency to accept information that affirms existing, familiar beliefs. New information that is different or unfamiliar is tuned out or rejected without any chance to be heard.

I saw confirmation bias thrive in fitness subcultures, including powerlifting, boxing, triathlon, and yoga groups. Confirmation bias can keep you doing the same workout for years or decades, independent of what's happening to your body. And you don't need to be a super fitness enthusiast to encounter confirmation bias. It can happen to casual walkers as well.

Be on the look-out for how you or the people around you are confirming and validating what you do without measuring and prioritizing health.

Another point: truth is not required for the brain to believe something is true.

Repetition doesn't only influence our associations; it also influences what we perceive to be true about our beliefs. The cognitive bias known as the Illusory Truth Effect is when we believe something is true based on how effectively (or emotionally) something is presented or by how often we hear it.

Why does this matter? Because repetition plus emotional experiences yields personalized truth and hardened beliefs.

The brain is lazy. It will take the shortcut to reaffirm what you do and know over the work required to learn and try something new. That's one reason why people like me keep doing things that abuse their body.

My advice? Start questioning your current beliefs and start measuring your health. And please start trying other types of exercises and give them enough time and reps to start believing in them.

Also, be aware of how the mind takes shortcuts in autopilot mode to validate and rationalize what you believe and do. If you aren't aware of how your biases are directing a lot of your actions, it will be harder if not impossible to change course in the name of health. This is true for exercise or for anything else that you want to change, including eating habits.

To learn more about the topics in this chapter as they relate to a major problem in your life or anything that you want to change, consider seeking out a licensed therapist. I'd also suggest the following books to become aware of how emotionally and instinctively biased our autopilot brains really are:

- *Thinking, Fast and Slow* by Daniel Kahneman

- *Habits of a Happy Brain* by Loretta Breuning

- *How Emotions Are Made* by Lisa Feldman Barrett

- *Blink: The Power of Thinking Without Thinking* by Malcolm Gladwell

- Lots of articles on any of the cognitive biases mentioned in this chapter

13

Why Habits Are a Bigger Deal Than We Think

Is there something that you do or don't do with regularity that you want to change? Eating less? Exercising more? Reading more? Fighting less with loved ones? If so, it's important to understand what the experts are saying about habits.[101] [102] [103] [104] [105]

Habits aren't trivial. They're a combination of emotions, psychology, people, places, senses, behaviors, rewards, and biases that develop over time and are unique to us all.

If poor eating, sleep, or exercise habits are part of your day, it's important to understand the fundamentals of habits first if you are determined to change. Why? Because about 40-50 percent of what we do every day "sort of feels like a decision," says habit expert Charles Duhigg, "but it's actually a habit."

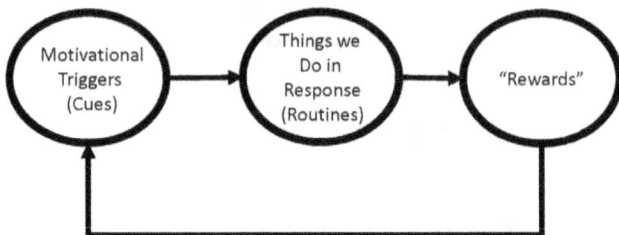

The parts of a repetitive Habit

The building blocks of a habit are triggers (sometimes called cues), routines, and rewards.[106] [107]

The triggers are one or more of what I call PPTTT concepts with context: People, Places, Things (sounds, sights, colors, smells, emotions, sensations, feelings, etc.), Thoughts (of people, things, etc.), or Times (of day) that makes you think of something you want (the reward) and the thing that you learned in the past (the routine) to get it.

For example, being in your car and getting cut off may automatically launch some cursing and yelling, something you may not do if you get cut off in line at the grocery store. Or you may not do it if your boss is in the car. Slight changes in the specific elements of the trigger influence the behavior. In this example, a change in context tells our brain to summon different behaviors or routines.

Why does this matter? Because changing anything requires a look at the triggers—PPTTT concepts linked in your associative memory—that launch your habits, whether they are exercise habits, eating habits, anger habits, stress habits, or whatever. When a routine is repeatedly launched in response to a specific PPTTT trigger in a specific context, it becomes a habit. A habit that gets launched in autopilot mode, often below the level of conscious thought. Unless you bring awareness to this automatic process, nothing will change.

I'd like to share how I deconstructed a habit that I never understood until learning about habits and PPTTT triggers. I'm someone who doesn't eat dessert a lot. I do have lots of vices: Fatty foods, salt, cheese, wine, chips, pretzels, and on and on. When I overeat or indulge, those are my preferences. Everywhere. Except, I always eat dessert in the homes of my mom and my aunt. These were the two homes where I was raised. Being in these places with these people, coupled with lots of great experiences for almost 50 years in these places with these people, launches a behavior that doesn't happen anywhere else. The PPTTT context is specific and unique.

If you exercise regularly, you likely have habits with PPTTT triggers like Wednesday at 6:00 is Becky's yoga class, or Tuesday is dead lift day, or you show up to the gym (the place) at a certain time and do the same elliptical workout (on the same machine or in the same area) at the same speed. These habits are linked to perceived rewards that are rated the highest to you in that specific context. If these habits are maximizing health, great. If not, bringing (conscious) awareness to the PPTTT trigger is critical to replace bad or build new habits.

Habit experts say this too: set small, incremental goals and don't try too much at once.

Just like overtraining a body part can result in injury or failure, we are set up to fail if we try to replace a lot of habits at once, diet and exercise. In that case, overload and quitting is to be expected. Do New Year's resolutions come to mind?

This is what tuning is all about. Setting incremental goals and working on creating mini habits with small wins within each tuning level.

Building a habit starts with consciously programming a trigger to do a planned routine and repeating it over and over again.

To build a new habit, start by picking a PPTTT (people-place-thing-thought-time-of-day) trigger that will physically remind you to do something. Triggers can be anything. Setting an alarm on your phone to do a predefined stretch once an hour is one idea. The trigger is the alarm, the routine needs to be planned, and the reward is feeling better.

Sitting hurts my body. I wanted to correct the effects of slouching forward. I made the doorway to my bathroom a trigger to do a back bend. At first, it took conscious effort. Now I don't even think about it. When I leave my bathroom, I do a stretch in the doorway for up to 20 seconds.

Other ideas for triggers: Leave out a yoga mat to do two minutes of breathing and stretching after your commute. Leave out a pan at night to cook breakfast in the morning.

To build a new habit, keep it simple by defining incremental goals (small wins), setting a PPTTT reminder, determining a routine, and doing it enough times to make it stick.

I found another fact about habits to be both interesting and essential in changing bad habits: The neuro pathways where habits are stored are hard coded in the brain and don't go away. But with reps, routines can be **replaced** to convert a bad habit into a healthy one.

Here's an example of a routine replacement: Mom or Dad come home from a rough day at work and a gnarly commute only to find kids, homework, and dinner prep challenges. That kind of situation triggers some junk food snacking (routine) to get the reward of lower stress (and dopamine.)[108] And it keeps happening.

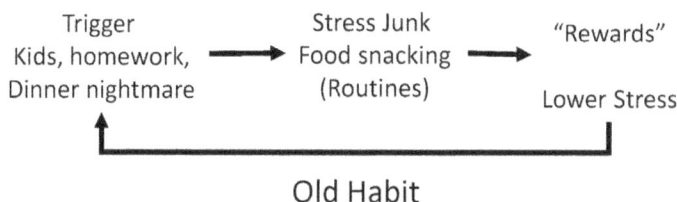

Trigger
Kids, homework,   Stress Junk   "Rewards"
Dinner nightmare   ⟶   Food snacking   ⟶
                         (Routines)   Lower Stress

Old Habit

But the routine can be replaced. If Mom or Dad catch themselves when the behavior is triggered, they can replace the bad habit with a new routine of breathing or yoga for a few minutes to get the same reward.[109] [110]

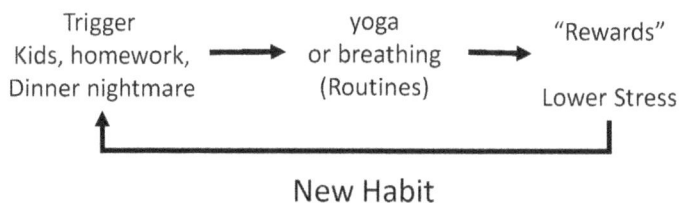

Trigger
Kids, homework,   yoga   "Rewards"
Dinner nightmare   ⟶   or breathing ⟶
                         (Routines)   Lower Stress

New Habit

Here's another example: I used to like hard workouts that made me sweat a lot and made me stronger. Cycling, boxing, and muscle isolation lifting gave me these rewards. After my fitness divorce, I read up on Pilates Reformer because I heard that it made athletes get stronger in new ways. Well, I tried it for several months and was sold.

My trigger to go workout was previously limited to specific workout routines. Pilates reformer workouts were a new routine that gave me the same rewards and strengthened areas where I was weak. It takes repetition to get good at new routines. But it also takes repetition to appreciate the rewards.

Understanding the habit replacement formula is important: Recognize the trigger and have a predefined alternative routine to get the same reward. Then build a new habit with repetition.

How will you measure, track, celebrate small wins? Answering this is important to make habits stick. It's important to track these incremental goals and wins.

When you meet a small milestone, it's important to celebrate it in some way that matters to you. It can be as simple as an affirmation or a piece of chocolate. (Just a piece.)

It's not common to hear about a fitness goal like exercising for 10 minutes for five straight days or eating breakfast for five days in a row. What is common? The end goals. I want to lose X pounds. I want to run a 10K or more.

Well, what happens after Week 1 with distant goals like this that aren't broken down into smaller wins? We still end up feeling far away from our goal, even after we did something positive. It's hard to feel good about positive incremental steps if we don't frame the larger goal as an accumulation of small wins.

Falling short of expectations[111] [112] also triggers the stress hormones in our brains, making the situation even worse. Yes, your expectations may be the source of your unhappiness and the root cause of failing to stick with a habit.

Remember social comparison bias from Chapter 2 where happiness and success are judged in relation to others? It's alive and well in all of us in fitness, to varying degrees. Ads and culture set high expectations but don't teach you to acknowledge and suppress this innate, always-on, social comparer in order to celebrate your achievements relative to your starting point. Instead, they stoke our social comparer by bombarding us with their aspirational reference points. Well, if you want to jump on a path toward better health, acknowledge and suppress this bias that keeps you caring about looks, performance, and social rewards more than health. Then surrender to where you are and learn to celebrate your small wins.

However, be careful about what you are celebrating. Remember that most of us are wired to "feel good" about rewards other than health. Some of our habits that produce unhealthy outcomes can be coated with hormones and neurotransmitters that can make us feel good. This is how people like me keep doing exercises that are bad for our body.

Oxytocin, for instance, is our trust chemical. It makes us feel good about a beloved instructor, gym, exercise group, or place. Leaving oxytocin-enriched exercise habits to diversify for health is hard. I learned this when I had to walk away from cycling and my personal boxing trainer—two great sources of this feel-good chemical.

Serotonin is our social comparison hormone. Anything that we do that makes us feel social dominance, respect, status, or importance gets a serotonin bump. I felt good from being able to do hard workouts, but we also can get serotonin bumps from winning, finishing, or improving. Feeling accomplished or better than others can be an anchor that prevents us from changing, when needed. I know firsthand that it's hard to embrace exercises perceived to be lower-level or things that you aren't good at if you have above-average abilities in fitness accomplishments that society cares about.

Endorphins from exercise also can make you feel good. They've been studied to improve mood and even decrease stress or depression.[113] [114] Runners often discuss a feel-good "runner's high." But if this "high" is making you prioritize running over health, especially if running or any fitness activity is known to be the source of injury, how is that benefiting your long-term health?

Happy chemicals can make an exercise habit feel good physically or emotionally. They are invaluable. Get as many happy chemicals as possible on your fitness path that is leading toward health. I want you to feel great from fitness.

However, and this is a big caution, if you are on a stale or abusive path, it's imperative to recognize that these feel good chemicals may drive you to keep doing the same thing. I kept doing unhealthy things to my body with exercises that made me feel good. Biases and habits aren't just mental. There is a physical component in our brain chemistry; an evolutionary nudge to keep doing the things that make the brain happy.

If our ancestors didn't push through a little knee pain or a sore foot to hunt and gather, we would be extinct. However, that's an example of ignoring pain for survival needs like food. Today, we ignore pain for esteem and aesthetics to our physical and financial detriment when we end up with pain and medical bills.

The bottom line: Habits are a big deal. Our habits are launched automatically, programmed with past experiences where health wasn't the preferred reward.

My advice: Start to question "feeling good" from fitness. It can be a rationalized excuse to not diversify toward healthier habits.

Also, start thinking about and deconstructing your existing and desired habits. Bad ones will keep getting launched automatically without intervention. Building new ones takes planning: program the trigger and put in the reps to make it automatic.

Consider seeking out a licensed professional who can help you address issues related to sleep habits, addiction, eating disorders, or if you can't figure out why you won't stop a fitness program that is hurting your body. I also suggest reading the following books for more information on habits:

- *The Power of Habit* by Charles Duhigg

- *Atomic Habits* by James Clear

- *Better than Before* by Gretchen Rubin

PART 4

Pivot Toward Your Health-First Fitness Future

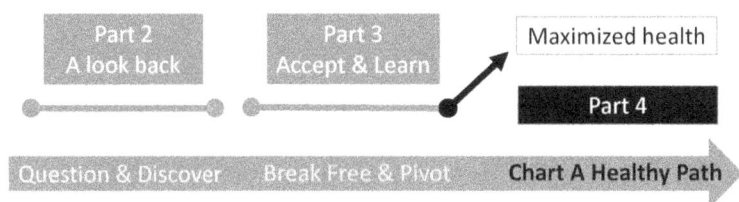

Anyone who has successfully changed an area of their life by themselves or with professional health knows that there are three steps: Accepting the influences of our past, learning skills to move forward, and then committing to taking the first few steps in hopes of building lasting habits.

If health is your fitness destination, and if you are like the tens of millions who have had fitness influences steer you away from it, it's time to start planning a new route.

14

Setting Your Goals, Your Club, Your Clock

Now it's time to build a plan. For fitness to be about you and your health, it's important to:

- Set new long-term goals based on what truly matters to you.

- Choose a teammate(s) for your new health club. Pick one or several people to share your plan and celebrate incremental, tiny health wins.

- Reset your clock. Take the time you need to build healthy habits from your unique starting point.

Set your goals. If your path is anywhere between slightly stale and really abusive, begin your pivot by linking rewards from fitness to what you truly care about.

When the motivation is about measurable health outcomes, you decrease the chances of becoming that friend, family member, or colleague you see living with pain. Plus, you'll have more money to do what you love with fewer medical expenses.

To help determine those outcomes, start by answering this question: why do you want a healthy body?

Habit and motivation experts[115] [116] agree that it's important to understand your motivations for change. Of course, no one wants unforeseen illness or pain, but do you really want health for the mundane things in life like binge-watching TV?

Why do you really want health?

Whatever the reason, make that your fitness goal. Make this your personal, intrinsic motivation. Don't wait for bad health to start caring.

To help answer why help matters to you, ask yourself:

- Describe the greatest possible day of your life that you want to live five to 10 years from now?

- Why does this day matter to you?

Close your eyes and play the movie of this day in your head. This should be the only fitness commercial that you care about. Who's there? What are you doing? Does it relate to a hobby, your religion, a dream destination, a vacation with friends, your family, or a reunion? Seriously, visualize it.

Next, ask yourself:

- Are you shirtless with people admiring your abs?

- Are people standing around you watching you crush a dead lift?

- Do the rewards preached by fitness ads and culture really matter that much to you relative to your other goals in life?

- When you think about this day, do you have a major structural health issue that you don't have now, something that could have been avoided with a different approach to fitness? Will your coach, your gym or the fitness company that you admire be there for you personally or financially?

- What if the thousands of hours you spent exercising caused this structural health issue, preventing you from fully enjoying this day?

Fitness should not get in the way of living a healthy life and enjoying your dream day, but it does exactly that for too many people who prioritize exercising for looks and performance over health.

Our actions represent our values. If you really care about health, exercise should be leveraged to give you the best chance to live out this day.

Your goal should be entirely yours, but I'll share mine to show how I've shifted my priorities: I want to be able to take a lazy, meandering walk through the streets of Paris with my wife until the day I die. I want this for many reasons. For starters, my wife is the most important person in my life. We both love architecture and great cities and Paris is one of my favorites. We love great food, wine, random walks, and unique, small businesses. Yes, my fitness goal unapologetically involves drinking wine.

Also, this is a goal because I'm a fan of corner, family-owned businesses because I grew up in a Chicago neighborhood with those types of businesses on every corner. They're gone now but they still exist in Paris. Finally, Paris was where Lorraine and I had our honeymoon and the place where I realized that I needed to end my broken relationship with exercise.

I know what I want out of fitness. I know that a little more ankle stability, better posture, and a little more strength and mobility in the center of my body will go a long way in taking that stroll in Paris years from now. That's why I focus on celebrating the improvements to my weak links. That's why I don't care if I'm the only man in some barre or Pilates classes. That's why I could care less if I can't finish a coveted social fitness goal like a 10K or that I have no clue how much weight I can lift anymore (because I know that maxing out or super-heavy lifting is not required for long-term health.)

You'll be surprised how liberating it is to make fitness about you. But first, ask yourself why you want health. Let that fuel your motivation.

Choose your teammate(s). Let's face it, celebrating is more fun when we do it with others. Habit experts talk about the power of sharing wins and goals with others.

Your new health "club" needs to consist of at least one other person who will team up with you on planning, building, and tracking your health plan.

When we share our workout plans for the week with a teammate and they do the same, our stated intentions carry a little positive pressure to follow through. Plus, a teammate gives you someone who will care about your small wins. The world won't care about your increased ankle stability or your ability to do one squat with great form. You know who will? Your teammate. And you'll care about their small wins.

After I divorced fitness, I became committed to doing exercises that I could not do. One exercise was yoga's Warrior III Pose where one leg is on the ground for balance and the other leg, torso, and arms are lifted parallel to the ground. After about four months of practice, I thought I had it, so I asked my wife to take a picture. I wasn't even close! Like, not at all.

I thought I was 90 percent of the way to perfect form but I was maybe 40 percent of the way there. We laughed. I didn't care. It was a positive moment because I shared it with someone who cared about the fact that I was trying to fix my health. It's moments like these that are powerful in building habits. You can and should have moments like this with your spouse, partner, kids, friends, family members, or coworkers who are also working on structural health goals that likely aren't socially coveted wins. You're in the same club with the same club goals. You're just at different starting points.

It's important to choose at least one teammate or group of teammates who:

- Share your values.

- Share their weak links and measurable health goals and plans.

- Celebrate incremental health gains with you.

Habits are easier when people share the same values. It's more important that your fitness teammate shares your priorities and beliefs than it is for them to have a high level of fitness ability or knowledge.

In fact, don't assume that a super exerciser or fitness enthusiast is the best teammate. I can tell you from firsthand experience that people with strong exercise habits and beliefs may be riddled with bias and a reluctance to change. This was me. I also know top-notch fitness pros who talk about health but they are obsessed with looks and performance rewards.

Your child, partner, coworker, or friend who has never exercised may be a better teammate than an avid exerciser who doesn't share your beliefs or want to focus on health first with you.

It wouldn't hurt to pick one or more teammates at work as well. If you spend a lot of time at work, it will be incredibly helpful to have at least one support person there to share goals, bumps in the road, and celebrations of tiny wins.

Everyone in your circle needs to have a plan rooted in measurable health outcomes. Remember that you will not be good at certain things. To be blunt: When you focus on your weak links, you may need to start over and struggle with basic exercises. I did. Your team-mate(s) may struggle too.

Not being able to do something is not a setback. It's a positive step to surrender to wherever you are. That's why a teammate that embraces measuring and starting over is absolutely necessary. Take a step back and learn together. Laugh together. Talk it through. You will advance. It just may take time. Just revel in advancing together but at your own pace.

For this to work, group members can't be upset when others advance faster. Remember one of the realities of the brain is that when we compare ourselves to others and lose, stress can be the result. Stop comparing and start sharing achievable goals and small advancements with your teammate based on your starting points, even when you are at different levels.

A loved one may be working on intermediate exercises. You may be working at a more basic level. A third partner, perhaps your child, may try to work on more advanced core exercises. Who cares if your incremental wins are different? You can still celebrate together. Welcome to the power of making this week and month about your mini wins instead of being shackled to extreme, end-game results glorified by ads and fitness culture. There's always something in it for you if you make it about you and where you are now.

Set up an "off ramp" with your teammate. Sand ramps sit at the bottom of hills for truckers who have lost their brakes so they can safely stop their trucks. These are planned. Determine your "off ramp" for days, weeks, or months when things aren't going to plan.

When you plan to go to the gym or do a specific workout and don't, what is your backup plan? How about having a few stretches or breathing exercises to do at home as a backup? Whatever the answer is, just don't beat yourself up.

When you have an abnormal week, like one where you travel, what's your plan? When things don't progress on certain exercises as fast as you'd like, what's the next move? Put that exercise on the shelf and find new exercises at your level.

Don't forget the kids, if you're a parent. Parents teach habits and priorities. Please teach your kids about fitness for health and make them teammates too. As dysfunctional as my body was and as much as I hurt, I never once thought to not exercise. Sure, having fun playing sports when I was young gave me the bug. But my Dad was the major influence. He took me skiing, cycling, played tennis with me, and brought me to his gym with him. I learned fitness as a habit through him, but I let ads and culture shift my motivation and goals away from health.

Parents teach kids to do their homework before they can use a device or watch TV. This teaches priorities. Parents can make kids prove structural health before they play sports for the same reason.

Where are your kids going to learn about the fundamentals of health, particularly the value of head-to-toe structural health, other than from you? If you can't objectively answer that question, perhaps you should become a knowledgeable source or get them to someone who is. Stop assuming they are learning it in sports unless you can validate that the coaches have the capacity to measure and assign head-to-toe, structural, health-based assessments and programs. (See Chapter 16 for how to get started.)

Finally, don't take all of this so seriously. It takes time to learn new things and develop new habits.

Laugh throughout the process. The world isn't coming to an end if progress is slow. Let go of any obsession with needing things tomorrow. Move on from the all-or-nothing cultural pull. Take your time. Laugh. Communicate. Enjoy.

Set your clock for evolving health. In rebuilding your fitness, there's one critical first step: Stop using time as a "results" destination and stop expecting fast results. Unless you've been given a medical reason to do otherwise, use the clock to create small, incremental habits and measurable health wins.

If you go in with a mindset that this is something that you want to do for the rest of your life, you can relax and let every week be about taking a small step forward. Every 60 days can be used to try to build a new mini habit. Then the next 60 can be about a new habit and mini win. Repeat. Repeat. Repeat. Over five years, those amount to a lot of new habits and a lot more health.

I found success in waves. I progressed with some exercises more quickly than others. I happened to have issues throughout my body. Some were more correctable than others.

It takes time to learn a new type of exercise and become proficient. It takes time to work on stress management. It takes time to develop good sleep and eating habits. If you plan on living for a while, you have time to build health brick by brick. Your temple won't be magically built in 60 days.

Is there a clock on how long you plan to love your family? Is there a clock on how often you want to get together and laugh with friends? These are healthy things with no clock. Your fitness relationship doesn't need one either.

Learn patience. Understand that you have a lot of muscles and ranges of motion that have limitations. It's natural to not get this at first because head-to-toe structural function is foreign to many of us. It's the same with learning a new language. You wouldn't beat yourself up because you weren't fluent in a year or two. Don't expect your structural health to be great or the exercises that advance it to work overnight.

It's not about a magical quick fix. It's about health.

15

Weight Loss Habits that Start with You

Though this is not a weight loss book, weight loss, fitness, and exercise are linked. Millions of us set fitness goals that revolve around weight loss, only to fail. Some of our failures can be linked to fitness marketing which has successfully told us that exercise is the weight loss cure. I had to let go of my beliefs about the role that fitness should play in weight loss and come to grips with why the "diet and exercise" narrative fails so many people like me.

I'm someone who has always had a lot of great exercise habits and an ability to burn more calories than most people because of my size and conditioning. I also know more than enough about nutrition and how to prepare healthy meals.

My eating habits from the time I wake up until the early evening have been super clean for decades: Lots of raw and steamed veggies. Fish. Chicken breasts. Avocados. Low starch (low glycemic) healthy carbs. Oats. Beans. Olive Oil. Nuts. Clean, whole foods.

None of these things helped me lose and keep weight off after age 42. Once five o'clock rolled around, all I felt was stress. I had terrible nighttime habits and ate excessive calories. I usually went on to have a bad night's sleep. Rinse, wash, and repeat. I didn't have a diet and exercise problem. I had a sleep and stress-eating problem.

It's absurd that our culture broadcasts diet and exercise as weight loss saviors without acknowledging the following facts:

- An estimated 80% of Americans experience stress,[117] to a greater or lesser extent.

- About 50-70 million people have some kind of sleep-related problem.[118]

- Another 40 million Americans suffer from anxiety.[119]

- More than 8% of adults suffer from depression.[120]

All of these issues can trigger unhealthy habits, including bad eating habits. Without addressing root causes like this, how will a crash diet make a dent in someone's weight?

Experts have shown that exercise is not the weight loss cure contrary to the claims of fitness ads and gurus. As Canadian obesity expert Dr. Yoni Freedhoff says, "[Exercise] is not a weight loss drug, and so long as we continue to push exercise primarily (and sadly sometimes exclusively) in the name of preventing or treating adult or childhood obesity, we'll also continue to short-change the public about the genuinely incredible health benefits of exercise, and simultaneously misinform them about the realities of long-term weight management."[121]

Just like the fitness industry gets you working out without talking about your body, it promises ways to lose weight without factoring in your starting point.

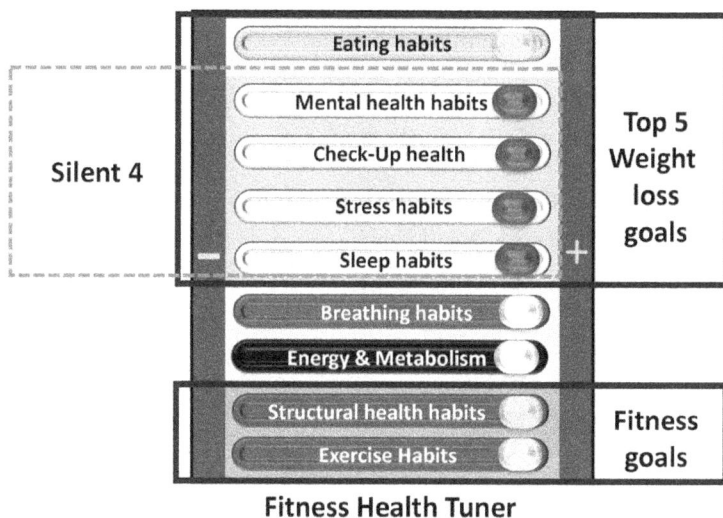

Fitness Health Tuner

This chapter is about sharing what I learned about weight loss in hopes of giving you a new perspective and a more holistic approach. I've found that:

1. There are potential health implications in believing that fitness should play a primary role in weight loss instead of a secondary role relative to the top five levels (see diagram).

2. The way most of us "go on a diet" is not aligned with a modern understanding of how to effectively build lasting habits.

3. It's important to consider your Silent 4 tuning levels in your approach to changing eating habits if weight loss is a top priority.

4. Breathing is one of the best-kept secrets for breaking bad

habits. It can help with weight loss to practice relaxed, deep breathing, especially if you are a stress eater.

The goal of this chapter is for you to begin thinking about how each level in the tuner impacts your weight loss goals and habits. This is how your weight management starting point starts with you.

To begin, please stop setting weight loss-related fitness goals. What? Yes. I just said that. If you want to lose weight and keep it off, stop depending on exercise as a primary tool in your weight loss tool kit.

I get it, exercise can burn a lot of calories for some people. If done in large or intense doses, it can slightly increase the odds of weight loss.

However, I'd like you to answer this question: do you believe that exercise should be a primary or secondary contributor to weight loss and weight maintenance?

A diversified exercise program absolutely can and should be a support player in weight loss and maintenance.

There are, however, some health pitfalls in believing that fitness should play a primary role in weight loss—something fitness ads tell us because they make more money when we believe it.

When you believe that exercise should play a major or primary role in weight loss goals, you open yourself up to the possibilities of:

- Keeping fitness goals perpetually shackled to looks and performance outcomes.

- Using exercise as a crutch to avoid addressing major health issues like stress, anxiety, depression, substance abuse, and eating disorders, among others.

- Staying on a stale or abusive fitness path because your favorite exercises like cardio or high burn routines are associated with the emotional reward of looking better.

- Not prioritizing structural health because many exercises that advance it are probably not rated as high as those linked to weight loss cures in your mind.

- Making today's workout about today and never making fitness about long-term health.

Some people do regulate their weight with a lot of exercise, often people in their twenties and thirties. But life changes and those people start gaining weight later in life due to injury, slower metabolism, and work and family responsibilities. These people don't have a plan because they used exercise as a crutch for decades and never developed healthy top five tuning habits.

So why don't you ask yourself:

How much do you rely on exercise to manage your weight? Is it working?

If it's not working, why do you continue to believe that exercise is the answer for weight loss?

If you believe it's working but your structural health is not considered, are you willing to measure and possibly change?

The top five levels, not exercise, are the places to focus on weight loss goals.

Stop going on diets. Did you lose weight by dieting in the past? Did you keep it off?

If not, you did not develop lasting habits—for your specific life, from your unique starting point.

Going on a diet defies our modern understanding of effective habit creation. First, many people don't put in enough time. Habits require repetition. Second, many people try too many changes at once. That's a recipe for failure.

A deadline commitment to go on a strict diet can be like reacting to traffic when an expressway is shut down for a president or head of state. It's temporary. Maybe your GPS offers a new route during the shutdown, but after the motorcade passes, your preferred highway route is once again automatically set by your GPS. That old route never went away.

Similarly, when the diet is over, your bad eating habits are still hard wired as neuro superhighways and ready to launch as soon as you are triggered.

As Ann Graybiel, the MIT neuroscientist who conducted the maze experiment (referenced in Chapter 12), explains, "We knew that neurons can change their firing patterns when habits are learned, but it is startling to find that these patterns reverse when the habit is lost, only to recur again as soon as something kicks off the habit again."[122]

There's a good reason why Alcoholics Anonymous teaches its members to avoid people and places that trigger drinking.

Similarly, you have decades of learned eating habits that can be kicked off by PPTTT triggers at any time. Building new habits is like learning a new route during major highway construction. You accept that your preferred route is not available for an indeterminant amount of time so you commit to trial and error. With enough repetition and patience, you find a replacement route that feels natural.

Here's an idea if you haven't had success: Stop linking numbers to weight loss goals. Instead of, "I'm going on a diet for X number of days to lose X number of pounds," say, "I'm developing new eating habits and taking as much time as I need to get to a desired weight of X. Then I'll use my new eating habits to maintain it."

The former approach tells your mind that it's temporary. The latter frames long-term thinking about habits being developed and used to maintain a goal. Seriously, are you really going to do zero carbs, zero alcohol, or whatever you do when going on a diet for the rest of your life? Then why start there?

Build eating habits from your starting point. Our lives vary in many ways, including the people with whom we live (and their eating habits), the number of candy jars near us at the office, the length of our commutes, our work and sleep schedules, our finances, our upbringing, our access to healthy and affordable food, and many other differences.

I'm not going to cover what to eat or the fundamentals of nutrition here. Nor am I going to cover the numerous types of diets. However, I'd like for you to consider replacing the concept of dieting by viewing it through a new lens of your eating habits. Specifically, instead of focusing on "dieting" as simply what to eat and not to eat, bring your awareness to:

- The small habits that you need to build as a natural part of your life (going through the process outlined in Chapter 13).

- And the bad habits, possibly with deep emotional links, that are running in autopilot mode and need to be recognized, deconstructed, and replaced.

The following are some questions to deconstruct and bring awareness to your eating habits.

What eating habits did you learn from your parents or other trusted sources when you were young?

Youthful experiences are powerful. These can have lasting effects on our eating habits. Did someone in your family teach you to eat quickly? Did you learn to finish your plate and then all of the leftovers? That was true for me.

I understand now that overeating tendencies are wired in me to this day. Look back to your own upbringing for any nervous eating, overeating, eating fast (not chewing), treating food as rewards (which may be linked to parental approval), habitual snacking at night or between meals, fast food habits, the amount of junk food in the house, or anything else.

Did your parents hate vegetables? Do you feel the same way? I know parents who pass their tastes on to their kids. Did your parents obsess about their weight or your weight and always talk about needing to go on a diet?

The diet books don't start with your psychological and habitual upbringing as it relates to eating. Bring awareness to your past to preempt triggers from launching unhealthy habits.

Are there people who currently play a role in your bad habits?

Is there someone in your life who triggers bad eating habits or is a codependent partner? Sometimes we share bad habits with positive people in our lives. For example, what if you and someone in your home both share the same habits of stress eating or drinking? Perhaps, you come home from work and talk about stress while drinking alcohol, smoking, or snacking. The person in your home (place), the time of day (night), and the topic of work (thoughts) that create a stressful reaction are part of the trigger that launches the habit. It is really important to understand how other people in your life trigger, enable, or support your bad eating habits. If other people are part of your bad eating, bring them in on the solution. I found it impossible to shift my eating habits without my wife changing with me.

Have you created a system so your healthy snacks and meals will be available when you need them?

If preparing or buying healthy meals and snacks does not become an automatic part of your life, it can be hard for good eating habits to endure. The reason? Bad food doesn't require a plan. It's everywhere. Healthy food does. If planning and preparing health food isn't a habit, bad choices will likely prevail. Put in the reps to build this critical habit. Part of it should include what you do and don't buy when you shop.

How do your eating habits earlier in the day, or previous day, impact subsequent eating habits?

It's really important to start tracking when you crash, feel sluggish, experience energy dips, or have cravings. Look at how bad eating habits later in the day can be linked to what you did and didn't eat earlier. Not eating enough food for breakfast or lunch all but guarantees overeating at night for me. Too much coffee in the morning impacts stress eating for me too.

Figure out the cause and effect of what and when you eat and how that has a ripple effect on your health and subsequent healthy or unhealthy eating habits.

The final question: perhaps what I call context restriction will work for?

I have switched from a belief in extreme diets with all-or-nothing restrictions like zero carbs or zero alcohol to PPTTT context restrictions. For example, there's a difference between sharing great wine with friends on a Saturday night and drinking average or crappy wine at home on a Tuesday because of a bad day at the office.

There's a difference between going out for cupcakes with your kid for a celebration than stress eating or emotionally eating cookies or cupcakes from the pantry because they're there. There's a difference between enjoying chocolate to reward yourself at the end of the week for something versus habitually eating candy from the office candy jar on a random afternoon. It's the same food or drink, the difference is the people-place-time-thoughts-things context.

I find that context can produce a different answer that you can ask yourself the day following bad eating or drinking: Did you enjoy it yesterday? I discovered that many of my "bad" eating, like having pizza on a Tuesday night because I didn't prepare healthy food, did not make me happy. In fact, it added stress. Alternatively, having pizza with friends and family on the weekend is enjoyable. It's hard to give up things that we enjoy, like "bad" food or drink wrapped in positive experiences. It's easier to give up "bad" food or drink wrapped in negative or "just because" experiences when we automatically eat, drink, or smoke things for no other reason than we never programmed an alternative habit to a PPTTT trigger.

I believe too much of the diet discussion revolves around labeling foods as good and bad. This drives people to unsustainable all-or-nothing restrictions. I think too little emphasis is given to autopilot habits related to boredom or negative triggers, including how things like stress, anxiety, or emotions like unhappiness or discontent create habits launched in autopilot mode with a specific PPTTT context.

Perhaps, you'll discover that the majority of your bad eating is done in PPTTT contexts where the experience doesn't really make you happy. There are diets out there like *Weight Watchers* that allow all foods into your diet. Perhaps, you can learn to incorporate them in moderation by considering restrictions related to certain people, in certain places, or at certain times of the day or week. For me, this made habits more sustainable than the all-or-nothing diet cycle.

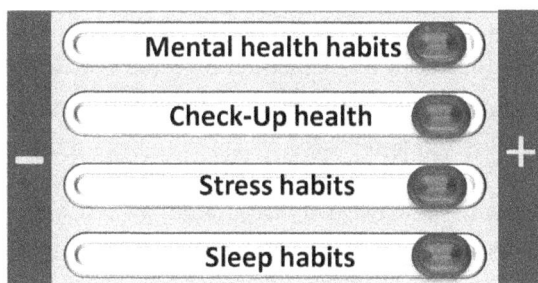

Silent 4 Tuning

Consider your medical health, mental health, stress, and sleep. In addition to expanding your notion of diet beyond what to eat and not eat to include how your past wired your autopilot eating habits, it's important to answer this question: What is the interdependency between your eating habits and how your Silent 4 levels are tuned? That may be the most important weight loss question that you've never been asked. If your eating habits relate to sleep, stress, anxiety, depression, or any combination thereof, starting a eat-this-don't-eat-that diet is probably destined for failure.

Start tracing your eating habits back to one or more of the Silent 4 root causes to begin making your approach to weight management about you. They are silent in most fitness ads, but they can have a noticeable influence on eating habits for many of us. They did for me.

If you have any negative tuning in these four levels, specific habit creation and replacement goals should be given serious consideration. This starts with understanding your Silent 4 habits and what triggers set off a chain reaction that leads to bad eating habits.

If you can't figure out how to deconstruct these habits or solve them on your own, please get some professional help. Also, if you have negative tuning here, please stop relying on excessive exercise for weight loss. All you're doing is punting a need for change down the road. You may even be focused on exercises that you believe are best for weight loss but are hurting your long-term structural health. I did this for way too long.

Get checkups. If you have health insurance, a good way to measure and track health is to get in the habit of getting a medical checkup. If you don't have insurance, I understand that it can be harder but try to look for free or affordable options. Use your doctor as a way to stop automatically presuming health from exercise and start tracking how specific types of exercises impact your health. Talk with your doctor about changing exercise habits and correlating them with your checkup results.

For example, perhaps adding some interval training can help your blood sugar levels or blood pressure if your doctor says that's okay. Maybe adding strength training positively tunes some levels like blood pressure or your lipid panel.

Perhaps, you can do high intensity interval training[123] or track your VO2 max if that test is available to you. VO2 max is a measure of the body's efficiency in delivering oxygen to muscles. Like lean muscle tissue, it decreases with age, starting about age 30.[124]

Checkups are also a great way to begin a change in eating habits with the goal of a measurable health outcome. Get tested in advance to see if a change in diet impacts your blood sugar, cholesterol, or other health indicators. Find a nutrition-forward doctor who is on the cutting edge of researching dietary methods, like time restriction, intermittent fasting, or intermittent calorie restriction to improve health metrics. I've known people who have successfully improved cholesterol and type 2 diabetes, for example, by working with such doctors.

The checkup will also help you understand if you have medical issues impacting your weight management. Also, ask for referrals to other resources like a dietician or psychologist if you need help building healthy eating habits.

Think about your mental health habits. Some people have habitual routines, running in autopilot mode in response to depression, anxiety, anger, sadness, or other negative states of mind. If someone has emotional eating habits, an eating disorder, or eating habits linked to depression, anxiety, or drug use (alcohol, marijuana, other), it is absurd to tell that person that diet and exercise are the solution to weight loss without looking deeper. There's also another link to depression and anxiety—joint pain. Yep, joint pain may lead to eating or drinking habits through depression or anxiety.

If you have any such issues, I suggest that you start by contacting a licensed professional. There are people who specialize in weight-related eating problems and other issues. Even if you don't have a "diagnosable" issue, you may have PPTTT triggers that launch feelings of sadness, anger, bitterness, or other negative feelings that lead to bad eating habits.

For example, let's say someone gets sad in the middle of the day and goes for an ice cream snack during work. This can impact their blood sugar levels and create cravings for bad foods later in the evening. Similarly, what if anxiety or depression lead to eating or alcohol consumption? This can negatively impact eating habits and sleep that night or the next day.

Start connecting the dots between how you feel, when you feel it, what caused you to feel that way, and what you eventually eat.[125] Get to the root cause and start tuning there.

Examine your stress habits. If you experience stress, that's not unusual. But have you ever deconstructed your stress related PPTTT triggers and habitual routines? If you have stress habits that result in bad eating, directly or indirectly, a replacement strategy could be invaluable for weight loss.

A direct stress habit is when stress launches the bad habit like excess eating, drinking (alcohol), smoking, or a trip to a candy jar at work.

Stress can indirectly influence bad eating.[126] For example, someone may be stressed at work and take the negative emotions with them on their commute. The stress gets worse, and they go home stressed and eat, drink, or smoke.

Don't discount stress as a first place to build or replace habits to change eating habits. Start recognizing stress PPTTT triggers and build replacement habits like doing breathing exercises[127] or 20 seconds of an exercise with deep breathing, calling a friend, going for a walk, or anything else that helps.

Review your sleep habits. I know firsthand how hard it is to suffer from sleep issues. Missing sleep has been linked to heart disease, cardiovascular disease, and kidney disease, among other issues. If you have them, it's important to take a serious look at your health and to understand specifically how bad sleep relates to your eating habits.

Bad eating or drinking impacts your quality and amount of sleep.

Alcohol, for example, is horrible for sleep. Missing out on sleep means your body produces less leptin—a hormone that make us less hungry—and increases a hormone called ghrelin, which increases hunger.[128] This is how bad sleep can be the link between yesterday's nighttime eating habits and today's bad eating.

It's important to learn how foods impact your sleep. Other than alcohol, things like fatty foods, spicy foods, and caffeine also can impact sleep.[129] Things like drinking too much liquid late at night can impact sleep because you need to wake up to use the bathroom. Finally, when we don't sleep, we have less energy to exercise the next day. All of the tuning levels are interrelated.

Start monitoring the answers to these questions:

- When you do sleep poorly, what types of food did you eat the prior day and when?

- Is there a connection between what you eat at night, your sleep, and what you crave the next day?

- Finally, are there other non-diet related experiences or thoughts that you can correlate with good or bad sleep?

Use devices like your smartphone or other wearables to track your sleep and get a quantitative view into the impact of eating habits on your sleep. Start researching sleep if you have issues and seek professional help if your issues linger. Sleep is not something to mess with.

Consider your breathing habits. Some may wonder why I didn't label this tuning level meditation habits. It's true. Some people can evolve breathing habits into systematic meditation habits. For others, meditation may not quite work for various reasons. I get it. It's personal.

But consider breathing for several reasons. For starters, breathing exercises have been linked to improved blood pressure, attention, control of emotions, and immune system health. Breathing exercises have been shown to improve focus, increase positive emotions, reduce stress, reduce blood pressure, and boost metabolism.[130] [131] [132]

Whether or not someone is ready for full-fledged meditation, breathing exercises should be considered health tuning for two main reasons.

First, you may love it and evolve your focus on breathing into an "official" meditation habit. You'll never know unless you try.

If meditation isn't your thing, the second reason is merely taking a few deep breaths helps with stress, even when you don't have a lot of time. It's such a powerful, cheap, and easy tool to slow down your day and your mind. Breathing is a way to bring awareness to and not react to PPTTT triggers. It allows us to consciously intervene and say no to things that are bigger in our head than in reality. Otherwise, our reactions can lead to a temporary fix, like nervous eating, smoking, or drinking for a quick dopamine hit.

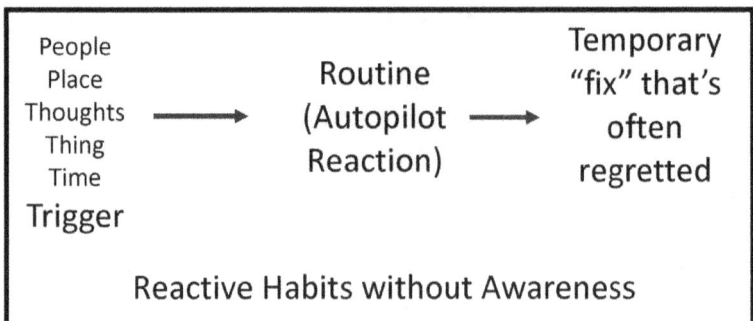

People
Place
Thoughts   Routine   Temporary
Thing   ⟶   (Autopilot ⟶   "fix" that's
Time   Reaction)   often
Trigger   regretted

Reactive Habits without Awareness

For my bad habits, I use breathing in the same way that the police use perimeter checkpoints when dangerous fugitives are on the loose. When necessary, cops shut down roads and highways and check to see who and what is inside each vehicle. Breathing lets you slow things down and take a look at what is happening in your head. It's a way to pull autopilot reactions off to the side of the road.

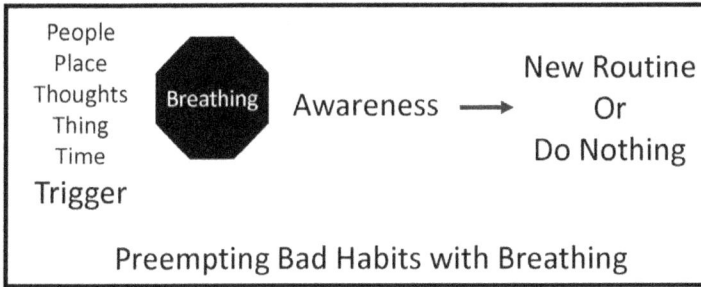

People
Place
Thoughts   Breathing   Awareness   ⟶   New Routine
Thing   Or
Time   Do Nothing
Trigger

Preempting Bad Habits with Breathing

This is what deconstructing habits and tuning all of the levels is about—becoming aware of your PPTTT triggers, your go-to reactions, and how your habitual reactions at each level impacts the other levels.

Try using breathing to bring awareness and acceptance to your bad habits as they are happening.

Try using breathing also as a habit replacement strategy to not react in the moment to stress, anxiety, depression, bad sleep, or other negative situations. It can give the same calming rewards that bad habits offer but it takes work.

Adjusting your energy and metabolism. I call this an "auto-tune" level because it adjusts automatically when you tune other levels. There is metabolic variability at an individual level based on things like genetics, age, size, the amount of lean muscle someone has, and aerobic conditioning when they start.

Give it time to work. It can be a problem when someone sets unrealistic expectations for losing weight quickly with a diet alone or a diet and exercise plan without understanding their metabolic tuning.

Set weight loss goals grounded in health. You set a goal in the last chapter related to why you want good health. Now extend that by picking a healthy reason why you want weight loss that has nothing to do with how you look. I'd be lying if I said that how I look doesn't matter to me, but my biggest motivation for losing weight was to help my joints and to finally start sleeping better. My nighttime eating habits were negatively impacting years of poor sleep.

Also remember, it's entirely possible to be healthy with some jiggle, a paunch, or some rolls. That's up to a doctor to determine.

Some healthy reasons for setting weight loss goals include:

- Better health results like lower blood sugar, blood pressure, better cholesterol, etc.

- Less stress on the joints doing everyday things like walking or during exercise

- More physical energy and less sluggishness with a healthier diet, which can lead to more exercise and help supports top five tuning

- Better sleep and waking up with more energy

- Less mental stress and anxiety

- Fewer bad moods

- An end to the cycle of feeling bad about eating poorly

16

Becoming Body Aware,
Focusing on Weak Links

We're here. Fitness is no longer about weight loss. Now we have a chance to make it about your health. Let's start with becoming aware of your body, from your toes to your head.

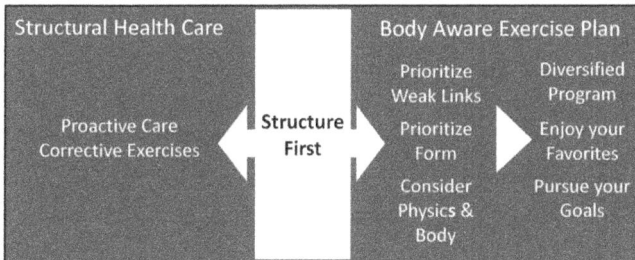

Structural Health Care		Body Aware Exercise Plan	
	Structure First	Prioritize Weak Links	Diversified Program
Proactive Care Corrective Exercises		Prioritize Form	Enjoy your Favorites
		Consider Physics & Body	Pursue your Goals

Recall our structure-first priorities: They reflect an approach to fitness grounded in body awareness, along with factoring in form, level, and physics. It's a framework that considers your body as the starting point.

This chapter will show you how to gain body awareness in one of four ways:

1. Getting proactive care from someone who is licensed or certified in assessing head-to-toe structural health.

2. Listening to your body.

3. Choosing places and people who help you become body aware.

4. Using exercises as indicators to track your body (moving a basic exercise or stretch from a "can't do" to "can do" list proves more stability and control of your body).

The first step is leveraging experts. The rest should be used as nudges to see these experts when you notice something is off.

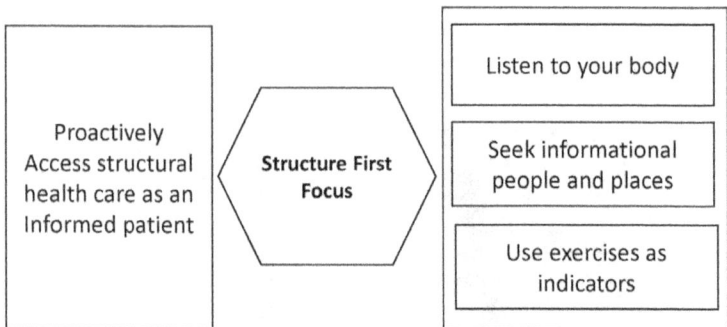

Proactively Access structural health care as an Informed patient	Structure First Focus	Listen to your body
		Seek informational people and places
		Use exercises as indicators

THE PATH TO BODY AWARENESS

Be an active, knowledgeable, and proactive client in the structural health care system.

Since all paths lead to getting help, let me share some tips that I had to learn after working with several therapists over the last six years.

[Note: This is not medical advice nor should it be taken as such as I'm not a licensed health care professional. It's a summary of things that helped me become an educated and proactive driver instead of a reactive passenger in the structural health care system.]

There are some things you can do before you go. Ask questions to select the right therapist or doctor. Ask how they test individual muscles and joints. Also, ask if you will leave knowing where you are weak, limited, immobile, or imbalanced (left to right or front to back).

Ask if their diagnosis procedure involves watching you move. Some therapists offered valuable, expert advice after watching me walk, balance, squat, and stand. I believe that health care of the future should involve a proactive checkup with an expert minimally assessing these basic movements, along with other joints tests and providing corrective exercises.

Make sure you have a full body assessment that includes chained patterns, like the lower chain from your feet through your hips. When I went to therapy for my ankle, I found out that my therapist could work only on my ankle. At the time, the State of Illinois limited my treatment to the areas of my body that were referred for treatment. Check and see what type of referral is needed to get you chain assessed.

Before you go, research to see if your therapist has expertise in your affected area and check for their continuing education experience related to your issue. For example, find an expert in running gait if you are a runner.

Go early and go often. Don't wait for acute, clinical symptoms to see a doctor or physical therapist. Make appointments for smaller issues like stiff knees, dull aches, or an imbalanced walking gait, even if there are no symptoms or pain. Who knows if one visit with the right expert can stave off thousands of dollars and pain in the future? Structural health care is far behind internal medicine when it comes to proactive care. It's likely that no one will ever direct you to seek care unless you have an obvious clinical issue so do it yourself.

Ask your doctor or therapist what they are testing and where you are weak, limited, unstable, imbalanced, or asymmetrical. Then write it down! You should make it a point to walk away with an analysis and readout of your issues, and you may have to ask them for it.

I asked a therapist for a diagnosis. He said upper cross syndrome, which among other things resulted in a weak lower trapezius muscle, which is critical for posture. I researched it, then looked up corrective exercises for parts impacted by the upper cross. I was able to do a lot of research on my own to become aware of my body and to try exercises to correct it.

Show them exercises that you can't do. They may not ask. I did a squat in front of one therapist. He simply watched the poor tracking of my left leg and prescribed physical therapy seconds later. Maybe you are better at lunging on your left compared to your right. Maybe you noticed in a class that your left side plank and right were totally different. Go to your therapist and show them why you think you are weak or imbalanced. A lack of left-to-right imbalance is something that an expert can assess. The fitness industry doesn't make a big deal about left-to-right imbalance. You should. Who knows how much you can correct it unless you try?

I cannot stress this enough: Shift the conversation from specific parts of your body to full-body patterns and your chain. It's important to learn how default changes are zigging and zagging up and down your body. Get your feet checked for a hip or lower back issue and vice versa. Ask if your posture relates to lower chain issues and what you can do to correct it.

In fairness to therapists, they may not bring up the chain because too many of us visit them only after a major clinical issue settles in. In those cases, they need to focus on the symptomatic area. Also, many of us don't complete a full round of therapy and leave before they can expand treatment to other areas. Don't stop therapy after symptoms decrease. Stop when you are aware of your weaknesses and you have corrected them or have a plan to correct them.

Seek out as many at-home exercises as possible. If you're therapist is helping you with symptoms but not giving you exercises to do at home, ask for a referral to augment your therapy. The best scenario is a holistic center that has multiple therapy modalities under one roof.

I found that therapy was great for detailed corrections. But exercises and stretches that I did at home, many of which I learned in therapy or from therapists online, are what restored the defaults in my muscles and joints.

I have a friend who suffered neck pain that he rated as a constant 6 out of 10. He learned to do two daily exercises, including a neck massage performed with lacrosse balls (the same ones used to play the sport). He went to an intermittent pain of 2 out of 10.

If you are doing something in therapy, see how much it costs for them to teach you how to do it at home. It's a way to get therapy every day, possibly without a huge time or money commitment. A balance board, foam roller, or balancing pad won't break the bank. Neither will lacrosse balls. Doing these exercises regularly at home can go a long way toward restoring good health.

Ask your doctor or therapist to be blunt about the risks associated with your favorite exercises, given the state of your body. You can ask something like, what might happen if I keep running, given my issues? I understand why doctors or therapists can be cautious about offering advice; many people are emotional about their exercise or sport. They may lose business because of patients' sensitivities, but it's important you know your limits.

Knowledge, care, testing, treatments, and assigned exercises (if needed) vary from therapist to therapist. I kept moving between therapists to gain greater awareness of my body. For example, three separate therapists assessed and treated my ankle with different techniques. They also assigned different exercises for my ankle and lower chain. I found value in playing the field.

Sorry if this sounds like a lot of experimental self-quarterbacking but that's how I had to do it. It's also how people I know finally got help.

My friend, Lisa, lived with agonizing, severe, sleep-impacting, deep pelvic pain after giving birth to her third child. It took her nearly four years and 13 doctors to get a diagnosis of "impinged femoral nerve." Treatment brought some pain relief but she created muscle imbalances in those four years. She then saw two more doctors, who recommended two more therapists to correct those issues. No success. She finally was referred to a therapist who diagnosed her pelvic and sacral misalignment. Among other stability and strength exercises, the therapist assigned two at-home corrective and alignment exercises. Two!

Those two exercises changed her life but it took nearly six years and 16 doctors to get there and correct the problem.

Find therapists who make you aware of your body and assign at-home exercises that make you feel good.

I'm sorry to be the bearer of bad news but an equivalent of the primary care physician for internal medicine doesn't exist for structural health care. Until you strike gold with the right diagnosis and appropriate corrective exercises, you need to be a vigilant self-advocate and navigate the system.

That's yet another reason why you should exercise for structure first and not let your fitness relationship incubate joint issues—to avoid this frustrating and expensive self-navigation process whenever possible.

Listen to your body.

There's nothing more important than paying attention to how your body feels, which you know better than anyone else. Then make a big deal about little things.

Considering your injury history is also a great place to star, it doesn't matter how long ago it happened. Find exercises with a trainer or someone in the health care system to see if you have basic function in a previously injured area and if an old injury has impacted other areas.

Other factors to consider are your aches and pains or stiffness after exercise. Tight hips, hamstrings, and neck stiffness can be signs of trouble. There are therapists, exercises, and stretches to fix this. Find out who and what they are!

Take particular note of how things feel different on the left versus the right side. My left always felt different than my right like walking and cycling. I never considered it to be a big deal. I should have made fixing that imbalance my number one fitness goal.

Take videos and pictures of how you stand and walk. You don't have to be an expert to see something glaringly different from one side to the other. Or a picture from the side can show bad upper body posture. If something jumps out, get to a therapist.

Don't self-diagnosis. Just look for clues to get to a professional for a diagnosis.

Do the same if you are a runner. Take a video from the side and back. With no formal training, I watch runners everywhere with glaring left to right imbalances and poor posture. Get to a therapist who specializes in analyzing running gait and offers exercises to correct it before you run again. This is what healthy, structure-first fitness is all about.

Choose the best places and people for body awareness.

Start judging your gyms, studios, instructors, personal trainers, friends, and "experts" based on how much they tell you about your body and help you advance at your level.

Here are some tips for choosing the best people and places for body awareness. The right ones:

- Offer classes or instruction with different ability levels and a focus on level advancement.

- Give great modifications after assessment.

- Focus on form fanatically and give corrections to the point of making you prove form prior to doing a class or starting something. (Note: There is nothing stopping a gym from posting a sign that says, "We care about health. We will comment on bad form." People and places who care enough to make you prove form care about your health.)

- Say no to you and tell you why—appreciate people who

make you aware of your body and don't let you exercise beyond your level.

- Explain how your assessment (physics, form, level, injury history, joint function) presents exercise-specific risks.

- Direct you to move in eight directions with a decent amount of time given to rotation and lateral directions. (Experienced trainers and instructors incorporate lateral and twisting exercises.)

I have exercised and taught at more than 10 different gyms and not one person said a word about my glaring left foot and posture issues that were visible from 50 feet away. Find people who can have a conversation about the head-to-toe chain, starting with the feet.

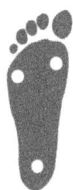

To take that one step further, look for instructors and trainers who are meticulous about foot form and upper chain posture, including the tilt of your head. Some exercises are taken to new levels when you focus on distributing weight through at least three points of contact—a concept known as tripod foot, as seen here—and become aware of weight distribution through your toes. When you focus on foot and upper chain form, you're not just correcting any weak links. You get the most out of your time exercising. For example, yoga's Warrior I Pose changes completely when you anchor the back foot with pressure on the outside and inside of the foot and when you activate your neck and upper back muscles.

If you can afford a personal trainer, it's worth it, even if you just go for a set amount of sessions to learn how to exercise with proper form. Seek out trainers who do continuing education on the mechanics of the body, not just classes to learn new types of exercises.

Trainers have varying knowledge of joint function. Ask them how they measure and track your body. If you are a lover of certain types of exercises like running or power lifting, it's worth your time and money to get someone to coach you on how to do it right. Stick with coaches who understand the joint mechanics and physics of the exercise.

Finally, please **stop taking unqualified advice.** It's everywhere in our I-do-it-so-you-should-do-it culture. If you want to maximize health from fitness, follow people who:

1. Assess your body and then tell you which exercises are right for your body level, physics, form, function.

2. Advise you on the long-term health risks and benefits of their recommendations.

3. Guide you to a way to measure health and when talking about joints, talk about head-to-toe chained structural health.

I believe that discussions on physics are much more important for high force exercises like running, jumping, and heavy lifting. Beyond total weight, limb length, torso length, and ratios of limbs and body parts can impact efficiency and stress on joints. Value people who can have these conversations with you about the types of exercises that you want to do.

In contrast, unqualified opinions:

1. Are given in broadcast mode with no consideration for what can make an exercise right or wrong based on your personal factors.

2. Claiming that types of exercises are "better" or "healthier" without directing you how to measure that.

3. Are given without knowing anything about how their recommended exercises impact health outcomes relative to an alternative, more diversified program.

4. Dismiss certain exercises without trying them.

If someone says exercise X is better than Y or is the best overall, ask how they measure "better" or "best" in terms of health outcomes for your specific body. Also, ask them if they've done an exercise that they are saying is inferior. Some people dismiss exercises that they can't do, have never done, or have tried very few times.

To me, it's clear: people or companies who advocate an exercise should know how to communicate risks and benefits for specific bodies.

Use exercises as indicators to track your body and create your running weak link list.

What's the easiest way to get the most health out of fitness? Focus on learning and doing basic exercises that you *can't do*. I'm not talking about benching 200 pounds or running a 10K. I'm talking about basic movements with just your natural body weight.

Why is this easy? There are hundreds of basic exercises that use different muscles, in different ways, with different dominant muscles controlling and stabilizing movements in different ranges of motion.

Why is this hard? We aren't taught to focus on things that we can't do. We've been taught to focus on things we know, things we are good at, and things where we are better than others. We were taught to value these rewards from a young age.

One of the biggest changes that is required to maximize health from fitness if you are on a stale or abusive path comes down to this advice (plea) from me to you: stop focusing on maintaining or advancing your strengths, including only doing things that are familiar or things that are popular culturally.

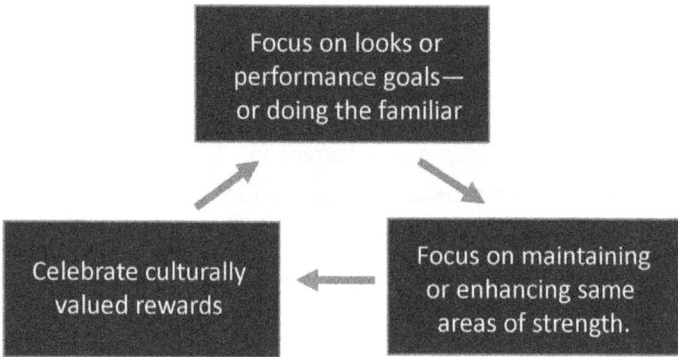

Focus on looks or
performance goals—
or doing the familiar

Celebrate culturally
valued rewards

Focus on maintaining
or enhancing same
areas of strength.

Stale or abusive focus
Not maximizing health outcomes

Make fixing your weak links your greatest priority.

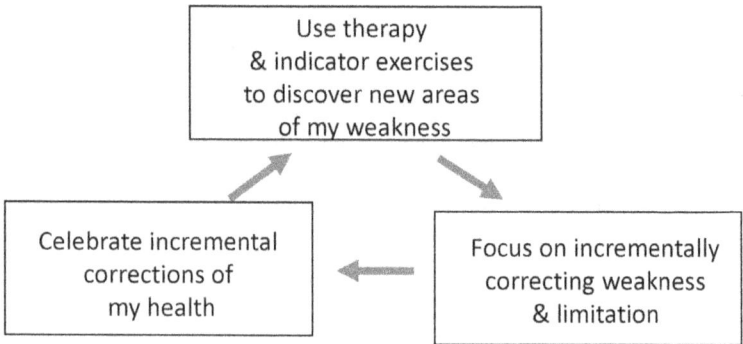

Use therapy
& indicator exercises
to discover new areas
of my weakness

Celebrate incremental
corrections of
my health

Focus on incrementally
correcting weakness
& limitation

Health focus
Maximizing health outcomes

It may seem obvious that learning new exercises can advance health but that's not how most of us spend our time.

In fact, I hope you are open to a belief that our huge structural heath problem is partially fueled by:

1. Too many people doing the same exercises too often.

2. A lack of fitness diversity.

3. A failure to correct weak links in general, and specifically before doing high force exercises.

If you want to experience the potential of your body, then I say: Break. These. Unhealthy. Habits. Start diversifying. Start discovering and focusing on your weak links.

Since 2014, I've been keeping a running weak link list—i.e. a list of exercises that I can't do in 10 reps with close-to-perfect form and at least 85 percent of range. I spent 100 percent of my time here when I first divorced fitness. Now I spend about 25 percent of my exercise time working on my evolving list of "weak link" exercises.

Your starting point and the state of your body should drive how much time you spend here. Those factors should also determine how much you need to stop or cut down on a type of exercise that negatively impacts your health.

I highly recommend that athletes and people who do high force exercises like running, sports, and heavy weightlifting impose a higher standard of joint stability and control on themselves, from head to toe.

Here is some general guidance for finding these exercises:

• Make sure they are at your level. See if you can do a few reps slowly—which requires more control and stability—through at least a quarter of the full range of motion with something that resembles about 80 percent perfect form. You can be a little off, just not a lot. If proper form is way off, find a different exercise at your level. Work your way up to doing the exercise for 30 seconds at your pace.

- Find as many single-sided exercises, also known as isolateral exercises, like lunges, side planks, balancing on one leg, etc. Testing one side helps brings awareness to your head-to-toe, left-to-right balance (symmetry). Make symmetry a big, big, big deal!

- Find as many exercises in as many ranges of motion for as many single or combination of joints as possible. This is how you test yourself and learn. Note that exercises with internal and external rotation of the legs and arms are some of the least popular exercises. Research some or hire someone to teach you.

- Take pictures and videos to know where you are and to check your form by comparing it to the proper form that you'll learn (preferably) from a trainer/instructor. Look for range limitations and wobbliness. Use this information to find small progressions for you to celebrate. Yes! Using your phone to track the evolution of your form and range of motion while doing an exercise is a cheap and easy way to measure the advancement of your health. It's also a great way to celebrate mini wins.

Where to start? If you can afford it, find a great personal trainer or holistic wellness center with people knowledgeable about the mechanics of the body and able to assess you. Qualified professionals, who know functional exercises that can test your ability to move correctly, are a great place to start, if only for a few times to learn how to exercise and expand your exercise repertoire.

A more affordable option is to explore the numerous exercises in Pilates and yoga that will test many patterns of chained muscles from head to toe.

After learning the specific exercises that are challenging for you, you can research these exercises and find out where your body lacks strength, stability, or mobility.

For example, let's say you can't do a high lunge in yoga. You can find a lot about a high lunge pose on the internet. You'll find that hip flexor mobility, glute strength, and quad (thigh) strength are required. Now you are more aware of specific weaknesses and limitations of your body. You can then find exercises at your level for hip flexor mobility and glute strength. Now it's no longer just a yoga pose. You have learned how this specific exercise is an indicator of your body's ability or inability to control and stabilize a specific movement with specific muscles. If you still have trouble finding out where you are weak or limited, get to a therapist or fitness pro.

I also recommend that you have an expert coach get you through the basics with a few private or semi-private sessions. You can even go with friends. For example, ask an instructor for a coaching session so you and some friends can learn form and the basics.

Pick yoga or Pilates to start and take your time to learn in a beginner's classes. Over the years, I highly recommend that you eventually try both yoga and Pilates and gain at least intermediate proficiency in each. Why? I have several reasons.

First, they are low force exercises with options at all levels. They also are natural body weight exercises. Once you learn, you can do them at home or in a hotel room—super cheap and highly accessible.

Second, there are tons of yoga and Pilates classes in gyms and studios, though yoga tends to be more available. Focusing here can help you build your weak link list for a while. Most of you can spend months to years here finding ways to advance your health by learning new exercises. There's no need to become a super-flexible yogi. Just try these exercises and see where you are limited. Don't worry about 100 percent range. Focus on getting as far as your body lets you go.

Third, these formats offer many single-sided exercises to make you aware of left-to-right imbalances. Yoga will test your ability to balance on one leg. More advanced yoga will test your ability to dynamically move in and out of a balancing position. Pilates will build core strength.

Finally, developing proficiency with yoga and Pilates enables you to build skills with low-force exercises that you can do for many years, even if you are no longer able to run or do heavy lifting. Many people stop exercising when they can't do their high-force, go-to favorites anymore. Proactively learn the low impact riches here, as early in life as possible. You'll prep your body for high-force choices while learning skills that you can do for a long time.

As one final note, I'm not just broadcasting "do yoga" and "do Pilates." I'm hoping that you discover new exercises with these formats. Then learn to do yoga or Pilates your way. I learned in classes and now I incorporate specific exercises that are good for my body into short workouts at home. It doesn't have to consume a ton of time. I'm hoping that you use yoga and Pilates in concert with great therapists and others in the fitness industry to find your weaknesses and limitations. Then you can focus on specific exercises to advance the health of your body.

Beyond yoga and Pilates, go alone or with some friends to hire a fitness pro to coach you through:

- Functional exercises

- Isometric exercises

- Exercises for (insert body part, muscle or issue)

- Exercises for (insert body part) mobility

- Exercises for (insert body part) stability

- "Core" exercises

- Scapular (shoulder blade) stability, strength, and mobility exercises

- Ankle and foot stability exercises

- Active stretches or stretches for (insert body part)—don't forget your neck, ankles, feet, and trunk rotation

- Strength exercises for specific parts that you found out to be weak in therapy

Also, if you have a gym membership, try new classes or new instructors. It's a low-cost way to learn what your body can and can't do. Whenever an instructor does an exercise that challenges me in different ways, I take notes when I leave class and add it to my list.

Finally, there's no reason to limit your scope of "cardio." There are lots of ways to elevate the heart rate other than running, walking, using an elliptical, or cycling. Boxing or kickboxing have more twisting and balance. There are even fast-paced yoga classes that elevate the heart rate once you gain a certain level of proficiency. Circuit training classes for weights are a great way to train your heart while working your body in eight directions (with a good instructor).

You can get your heart rate up with light weights and bands and do workouts where you are also working on strength, stability, and mobility. A lot of places also now offer high intensity interval training. If your doctor or therapist says yes, go for it. You can combine strength and interval training.

Health happens when you try new things and learn how to control and stabilize new movements. That is way less likely to happen if you have weak links and do the same exercises time after time that either don't correct them or make them worse.

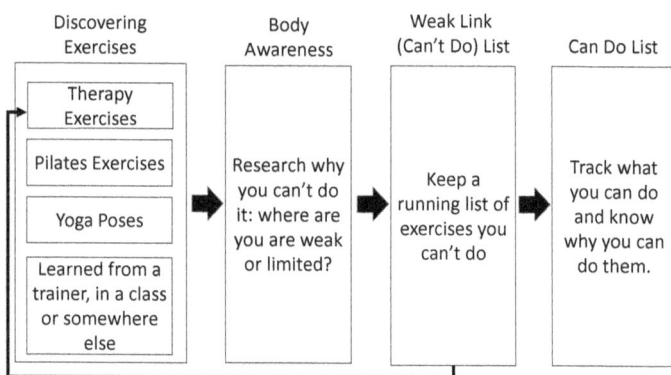

Discovering Exercises	Body Awareness	Weak Link (Can't Do) List	Can Do List
Therapy Exercises Pilates Exercises Yoga Poses Learned from a trainer, in a class or somewhere else	Research why you can't do it: where are you are weak or limited?	Keep a running list of exercises you can't do	Track what you can do and know why you can do them.

BODY AWARENESS AND CORRECTING WEAK LINKS

Find your "can't dos." Build your weak link list!

Learn why you can't do them via an expert or via research.

Why? It makes you aware of your body!

Work on exercises where you can't control and stabilize basic movements. Keep track of them. Over time, you will start moving more and more "can't do" exercises to your "can do" list. This is proof that you are advancing the health of your body, and it's a great way to track and measure your structural health.

This process allows you to expand your exercise knowledge and build new workouts from your ever-expanding "can do" list. Just keep in mind, if one exercise or body part does not improve, go back to your doctor or therapist and find out why.

Include time in a weekly program to focus a little here or a lot there each week. The more structural health issues you have and the bigger they are, the more time you should spend on them.

And please learn from my mistakes: Structural health may not heal if you keep doing the same things that are causing the issue, even if you do therapy and corrective exercises. For example, if running is negatively impacting your knees or feet, adding yoga once a week will likely not take care of the problem.

Take time off to focus on structure first. Walk away from exercises that hurt your body, even if you love them. Trust me, you can build up a new love for new exercises if you give them a shot. The notion of more fish in the sea doesn't just apply to romantic relationships, it applies to exercises as well.

Structural health takes work…but it's finally about you! I get it. There is no mass cure or workout. There is no nationally approved joint test that you can access at gyms with personal trainers. There is no standard entry point into the structural health care system or standardized head-to-toe test. That's the bad news.

The good news is that you can change the trajectory of your health if you find the right people to assess your body and the right exercises to correct your weaknesses. I didn't write this book to share a magic cure. I wrote it to share a realistic approach that I had to learn on my own.

You have to experiment to learn where you are weak and which exercises correct your weaknesses. If you have a bad or unsupportive experience along the way, try somewhere else. I kept taking my money to new places until I found people who knew what they were talking about. They're out there.

Eventually, something powerful will happen when you look at your "can do" list: You will physically feel how much you have accomplished by correcting weak links as a first priority. This will make you a believer in exercising for health outcomes. Feeling is believing.

17

Building A Complete Program That Starts with You

By now, I hope you've chosen your fitness teammate. This is the person with whom you will plan, measure, and track health outcomes in your new, exclusive, and deeply personal health club.

Time is not used as a destination. It's used to incrementally build habits and celebrate micro-advancements in health.

Weight loss goals are separate from fitness goals since fitness will be only a support player in weight loss. To lose weight, you'll figure out how to incrementally tune the top five levels and use breathing where possible.

Your long-term goal is set, and it's about why you want health. If you haven't done it yet, it's time to do it now. Write down your dream day that you want to live a decade or less from now. Write down the things that matter most to you.

This is why you want health!

This is your fitness purpose.

You're in the process of learning about your weak links and exercises that correct them.

And you've adopted a structure-first code.

It's time to tune your bottom tuning levels with a plan for your body that supports your goal. The plan will be separated into a weekly plan, a 60-day plan, and a six-month goal.

Why all three?

First, it's great to use every six months as a checkpoint period to diversify, measure, and recalibrate. If we never stop and pause, you can look back three years from now and realize you did the same exercises in the same way the entire time.

Second, habits require repetition to take root. Sixty days is a good time period to build new habits and to experiment with new activities. Maybe these 60 days will focus on doing five minutes of stretching at night. Or over the next 60 days you will try yoga once a week. Perhaps, you'll try a new class or hire a personal trainer one day a week for 60 days.

It could be a fitness habit plus another habit in the top five. Just don't try to do too many at once.

Finally, the weekly plan is about setting incremental goals and weekly plans with small wins that are shared and celebrated.

Write down your measurable health outcome goals for next six months and answer this question: over the next six months, how will I measure, track, and advance or maintain this health outcome?

I realize that the question includes the words "advance or maintain." I really want you to focus on advancing your tuning levels, including your structural health, not just committing to doing the same things. Too many people stay in stale relationships by not trying new things.

Here are a few ideas to help you answer the question:

First, your answer shouldn't be related to weight loss. That's top five tuning. The goals here are realized specifically via structural health and exercise habits with a focus on structure first.

Until you don't have weak links, as measured by doctors/therapists or by achieving intermediate proficiency in yoga and Pilates, a structural health goal needs to be on the list.

Your measurable health outcome goal at six months could include:

- Fixing a clinical weak link like left-to-right imbalances or a part that is immobile, weak, or unstable.

- Getting a stronger muscle, having better posture, or fixing tight areas of your body.

- Working specifically on exercises that focus on stability muscles like rotator cuff muscles, gluteus medius, inner thighs (adductors), or lower traps (trapezius).

- Moving a weak link exercise from your "can't do" list to your "can do" list is a great goal.

You can measure exercise progress with:

- Time. For example, you can count how long you can do an exercise like balancing.

- Quality reps. For example, perhaps you have an exercise on your "can't do" list that you track, starting with being able to do one quality rep and advancing from there. Video can help. Less wobbling and more alignment are great signs of improvement.

- Number of workouts. You can measure these based on how often you do something new like yoga, Pilates, or something else.

- Range of motion. Take pictures and videos to see how much more range you can get into exercises like a lunge or how straight your arms are in a (yoga) chair pose.

The important thing is to find a way to set a goal and track progress.

Other measurable health outcomes that you want to improve or maintain from exercise habits could include:

- Exercising for X days per week and Y time per day.

- Improving or maintaining heart rate conditioning. For example, perhaps you set a goal to walk with your heart rate at 110 beats per minute. You can research devices to measure your heart rate and talk to a fitness expert on a good target for you based on personal factors like age and conditioning level.

- Improving a checkup metric like blood sugar, blood pressure, VO2 max, or another issue that you discuss with your doctor or fitness expert.

- Being able to make progress or complete a type of class where you are learning something new like swimming, kickboxing, or yoga.

- Feeling better, as long as "feeling good" isn't an excuse to keep doing something that hurts your body.

- Working on form for a BBFSL goal with your physics and function in mind.

Next, write down specific focus areas for the next 60 days. The last step was your goal. This step narrows your focus to what you are doing to support the goal. It also allows you to create the repetition needed to build mini habits.

You may discover a lot of weak links and exercises that you can't do. There may be lots of exercises that you haven't tried. There also may be a lot of exercises that you know how to do. Maybe not. It doesn't matter. The clock is thrown out.

Use the next 60 days to learn and advance just a few things. Don't try to accomplish too much too fast.

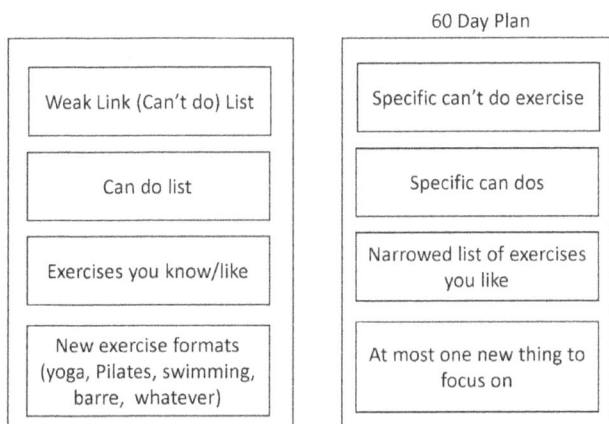

	60 Day Plan
Weak Link (Can't do) List	Specific can't do exercise
Can do list	Specific can dos
Exercises you know/like	Narrowed list of exercises you like
New exercise formats (yoga, Pilates, swimming, barre, whatever)	At most one new thing to focus on

There are four "lists" from which you can build your plan. The first two were from the last chapter: Keep running lists of exercises that you can and can't do and understand which muscles are used. You can also write a list of exercises that you know and like, including cardio. If your form, function, and physics are checked, put some of those on your 60-day plan.

Read up on common injuries or common weaknesses related to these exercises. It's easy to find data about the structural benefits and risks of exercises like running, biking, swimming, squatting, dead lifting, etc. There's also a lot on form.

Of course, researching information on the internet is risky. If you do an exercise frequently, the best approach is finding a coach or trainer that is knowledgeable in the mechanics of the body who can assess you. If you have lower chain (feet through hips) weaknesses or instability, a time out from cardio to focus on structural health corrections could go a long way.

Finally, I believe that you maximize health when you learn and try new things. The body gets used to repetitive workouts. Put something new on your list, even if it's a new instructor who does a familiar type of exercise a little bit differently. But only try to learn one new thing at a time. You'll have time to try other things in upcoming 60-day windows. Learning yoga and Pilates should be on this list until you get up to an intermediate level. They are great tests of structural health! Or pick types of exercise assigned by a trainer as long as you know how it relates to head-to-toe health.

Be realistic about your level and where you are with fitness habits. For example, do you currently exercise 45 minutes a day or is it zero? Do you do a lot of exercises with good form? Or are you someone who just does cardio and doesn't really have a background in strength or mobility training? Wherever you are, don't sweat it. Just start setting realistic goals that reflect what you can realistically do in terms of time and ability.

Perhaps, you currently don't exercise at all and a major victory would be exercising three times a week for 10 minutes. Pick a few exercises from your "can't do" or "can do" list that can be done in that time.

Don't discount the power of going to physical therapy as a first step. Find exercises there and focus on mastering those, plus maybe a few more that work to correct your weak links.

Pick at least four "can't do" exercises to work on over the next two months. Focusing on four exercises a week for two months is not major time commitment.

Perhaps, you can pick more than four and focus on different ones during specific weeks.

For example, if you had as many as 24 exercises on your list for two months, you can do six of them on weeks one and five, six on weeks two and seven, etc. It's all about diversifying and using your exercise time to work as many patterns of muscles as possible instead of overusing muscles by doing the same exercises. I tend to keep a list of 20-30 exercises that I want to advance in a two-month window, focusing on a few each day.

If you don't have them as part of your program, balancing and eight-direction exercises need to be on the list. Yoga, Pilates, kick boxing, Tai Chi, barre, and some dance and functional exercises that work on rotating or twisting are great for working on joint mobility.

Spend your 60-day windows looking for the good instructors and trainers who will constantly test your body in a lot of different ways.

Create a list of at least two quickie exercises, self-massages, or stretching that you can do during the day to make your body feel better. I call these Motwecs—move for 20 seconds—and Matwecs—massage for 20 seconds.

The 20 seconds part is not gospel. You can do these 20 seconds. You can do them for two seconds. Sometimes I do them for up to 10 minutes while watching TV. The time doesn't matter. What matters is creating mini, quick habits that can give you a mini correction and make you feel better.

If you don't know where to start, a therapist's office is the best place. Alternatively, look through the final part of this book at the list of exercises that I want to do for life. Doing things like seated figure-four stretches a few times a day can really help your health.

Let me share a few. I'm always working on posture, for instance. When I stand up, I clasp my hands, lift them up straight and do a back bend for a few seconds. I have many self-massage exercises that I've learned with the foam roller and massage (lacrosse) balls.

I often do yoga's Warrior I Pose for a few seconds. It's a great full body wake up. I regularly do a few wall angels (also called wall slides) to wake up my upper back and shoulder-blade connected muscles. I also do side rotation neck stretches, side tilt neck stretches, and chin tucks regularly. Doing just 10 seconds is a huge relief.

Learn the exercises and stretches that make you feel good! Do them for a few seconds. It can change your health if you find the right exercises for you.

I believe we should all understand specific exercises that we can do quickly, throughout the day that give us mini corrections. Therapy is a great place to learn. You can also find other reliable sources for topics like "stretches I can do at my desk" or "exercises for people who sit a lot." There's a ton of information out there.

These quickie, corrective exercises are among the most important things you can do in fitness. We always talk about needing to work out for an hour, 30 minutes or even for 10. However, regularly doing 10 seconds to a minute of an exercise that is meaningful to your body throughout the day can change your health.

The next step is to create your plan for the week. You've narrowed your focus for 60 days. Now write down this week's plan and share the plan for the week on Sunday or Monday with your teammate.

Your weekly plan should involve answering these questions:

- What are you planning to do this week?

- How often are you going to exercise?

- How does each workout map to a health outcome?

- Where will you do it?

- What is your PPTTT reminder? Is it a reminder on your phone or something else?

Pick a few items on your list of "can't do" exercises from your 60-day plan or from those assigned by a therapist. If you're like me and have a long list of "can't dos" that you're tracking, then pick the specific ones that you'll work on this week.

To help set your weekly plan, consider:

- Can you try a new exercise format? If so, where and when are you doing it?

- When, how often, and where are you going to work on breathing habits? What is your PPTTT trigger?

- Which Motwecs or Matwecs are you going to work on, and what is your PPTTT trigger? When you get home from work and change your clothes? After you get back to your desk from lunch?

- If you are sticking with your favorites, have you figured out a way to diversify during your weekly plan?

- What is your plan to elevate and track your heart rate? Are you doing the same-ole thing or are you trying different ways, like an interval strength training class, to "do cardio?"

Think about the body parts that are worked, and make sure you are working from head to toe. Rotate. Twist. Move left to right! If you aren't exercising in eight directions, it's not a full body program.

Don't forget to plan the celebration and rewards. Create your weekly and 60-day plans with measurable goals as granular as possible so you can celebrate the goals with your teammate(s).

This step is even more critical for those who "hate exercise" or feel like they "tried before and failed." People who feel like this need to find things to celebrate because fitness hasn't been a source of success in their past.

Celebrating the small stuff motivates us to believe in the big stuff. This will only work if you and your teammate care about the small things, like a little bit more hip mobility or a little more balance. To repeat: The rest of the world likely won't care. Your teammate will. Define and celebrate small stuff with your friends and family.

Plan your daily rewards when you do something.

Be proud of every workout. Celebrate every extra inch, rep, or second of advancement per exercise. Some will come faster than others.

Make sure you share your workout success with your teammate. Congratulations from a teammate is a big deal. Call or text but communicate. This is super important for people who have had negative experiences with fitness in the past.

What do your weekly celebrations look like? Fill in this sentence:

If we meet weekly milestones, we will _____ (fill in the blank). Minimally, a good milestone is just to sit down with your teammate or call each other and talk.

This will begin to make exercise about things you care about and can share that aren't superficial social rewards.

These 60-day celebrations are a big deal. It can fuel your motivation to set new goals for the next 60. In fact, bring your new milestones for the next 60 to the celebration. It helps reset your focus and keep the list of weak link exercises growing.

If your exercise program alleviates pain or takes control of your body to a new level, this is something to truly celebrate. Plan that celebration.

When my knees stopped hurting, I learned to think about fitness in a new light. When my hip popped less, I literally felt a correlation between that symptom being gone and a never-before-felt level of strength in the center of my body. When I found exercises to make my neck pain go away, that was a great feeling.

You'll feel these personal rewards if you set health outcomes as goals, value them, and then feel the benefits of exercising for your body. Celebrate!

Be sure to plan for setbacks with a specific "off ramp" plan. Have an alternate plan if you couldn't do the planned workout. Maybe you can do something fitness or non-fitness related that is positive.

Go for a quick walk if your body is up for it. Do a super-modified and short workout, like one or two minutes of yoga. Play catch or goof around with your kids. Practice a hobby. Do some breathing exercises for a few minutes. Other activities are okay if they pass the health sniff test—i.e. sitting in a park, breathing, painting, looking up healthy recipes, or even watching TV doing stretches, self-massage, and movements that make you feel good.

Find a new routine to follow after a stressful trigger or for times when you just don't want to exercise. It's okay if you don't feel like exercising. Just prepare a routine and reward instead of letting your brain launch a bad habit in autopilot mode. If you don't consciously prepare, autopilot default routes will prevail.

Also, plan for times when people in the fitness industry won't know how to make exercise about your level or body. This has happened to me a lot as a statistical outlier in terms of height and weight and as someone with lower chain issues. Don't let that get in your way. Find new people and places to support you.

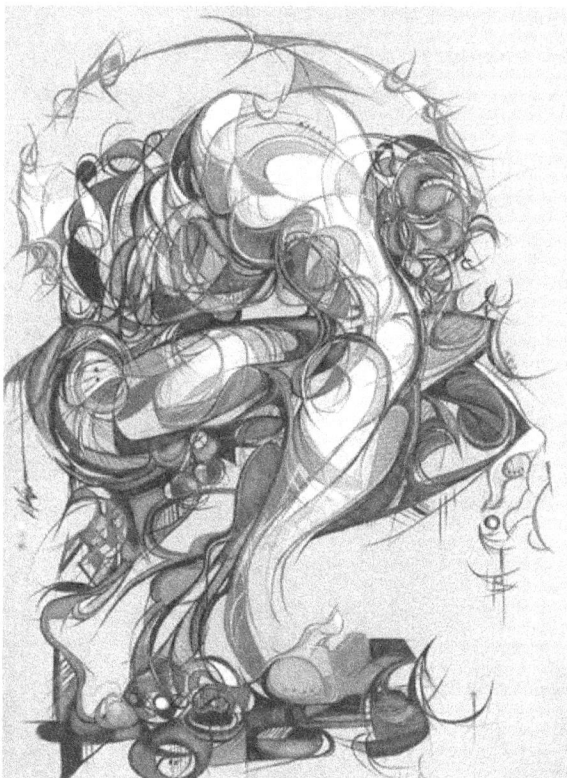

Remember this painting? It's called *Surrender to a new Beginning*. Shortly after seeing it, I asked the artist, Michael Korber, if he had back pain because of the concentration of barbs at the lower back and neck of the figure. In fact, he is riddled with pain from sports and exercise choices that he made before his forties, including heavy lifting and martial arts. That's one of many reasons I felt connected to him, and I've remained connected to the painting and his work ever since.

Take note of something else that is subtle in the painting. The figure is letting go of something. We often need to let go of something before heading in a new direction. Often, the thing we need to let go of is a problem of our own creation. It can even be something that we value or enjoy, even though it's not good for us.

Some of us wait until an injury gives us no choice but to let go of our fitness past. I hope that you don't wait for a serious structural health issue to finally make your fitness path about you, your health, and what you truly care about—now and in the future.

Isaac Newton taught us that a body in motion stays in motion unless acted upon by an opposing force. I hope you now realize that a body in motion with weak links, bad exercise form, and a one-dimensional program is likely to remain weak or get weaker, unless you act with common sense.

The path from where you are to better health is one worth taking. Do the unfamiliar and hard, not because it's socially glorified but because you're focused on preserving your body. Share that journey with people and let them share with you. In doing so, you're giving yourself the best chance to live a life that matters to you.

With incalculable appreciation for your time and my greatest wishes for your improved health,

Todd

PART 5

Exercises for
Today, Tomorrow &
the Rest of Your Life

Though I want you to find the specific corrective exercises that will work best for you, I'd also like to share my own list of exercises that I learned to use as indicators. These are the ones that I want to be able to do for the rest of my life.

This combination of natural body weight exercises tests my head-to-toe health and requires:

- Left-to-right symmetry

- Foot and ankle function

- Lower chain function

- The entire core

- Patterns that enlist a chain of muscles from the foot through the core (and across the body)

- Muscles and patterns that matter to upper body health, including muscles that connect to the shoulder blade

- The strength of the big muscles and stability muscles

- The mobility of my joints from head to toe

- How life and fitness programs are or are not advancing my structural health

I come back to these basics, which I was not able to do six years ago, to continually monitor awareness of what my body can and can't do.

You can use this list as a reference and to augment the program that you build with your trainers or therapists. I've included this list as a sample of how a combination of exercises and movements can test the body in different ways.

The second set of exercises includes harder ones that are indicators of a higher level of head-to-toe function if you want to reduce risk and increase performance in high force exercises and sports. This is also a list of exercises that parents can use with their kids to start a discussion about structural health. I'm also sharing these harder exercises as ways to require a higher level of mobility, control, and stability.

For all of these exercises, the best place to start is by hiring a personal trainer, yoga instructor, or Pilates instructor to walk you through the basics. You'll get feedback and, hopefully, they'll give you suitable alternatives as needed. I recommend that you try a group session to learn the basics and have an expert assess your form.

Finally, this chapter does not qualify as medical advice. Do these exercises at your own risk, and your ability to do them is not a guarantee of good health. It represents a series of exercises to explore and become aware of your body. Consult licensed therapists and doctors who provide assessments before you start. Begin slowly, and do not push past your ability. Stop immediately if you experience any pain or serious discomfort.

DO NOT push your body too far with any of these exercises. I use the "easy plus smidge" rule. Move into a range that is easy for you, and then just try a smidge more. That's your range. Don't force movement beyond this, your natural range.

You do not need extreme flexibility or 100 percent range of motion to become body aware. In fact, being limited to 10-60 percent of range is where you can become aware of a weakness or limitation. For example, I wouldn't be overly concerned if you are close to touching your toes while bending over in a forward fold (bending over with straight legs).

I'd make mobility of pelvic-connected muscles like lower back muscles and the hamstrings a top priority if you are far from touching your toes. The purpose of using these or other exercises and poses as basic indicators is to see if you are limited in your range, experience any pain while moving slowly, or have a lot of wobble or instability. This can indicate weak muscles, joint immobility, joint instability, or all of some combination thereof.

Here are a variety of exercises you can easily find online. Keep in mind that they test different muscles and be sure to focus on proper form. At no point should you feel any pain doing any of these, even if you are doing them slowly. Seek expert assistance if necessary and be sure to consult in advance with your health care provider if you are concerned about any issues.

Get your camera out whenever you can. Have a friend or partner take pictures and videos to check your form and look for any imbalances that may require therapy. Then show the pictures or videos to your therapist and ask for an assessment.

Also, please (times infinity) have an imbalanced gait checked and corrected by your health care provider or other professional. I know that some of us will always have imbalances for various reasons but that doesn't mean that we should give up on trying to improve our lower chain.

FOUNDATIONAL EXERCISES

Lying or Seated Figure Four Stretch: Try this exercise to focus on deep high rotator mobility and general hip and low back tightness. It's something you can do on the floor or in a chair during the day as a quickie stretch. Keep proper spinal alignment while leaning forward but look for other hip rotation and hip mobility exercises if this is too challenging. If this is really hard or proves asymmetrical for you, seek help from a therapist.

Single Leg Balance: This exercise tests the stability of your lower chain, one side at a time. Balanced weight distribution through the foot is a must and don't do it on the outside or inside of your foot. Distribute weight through the foot and make sure there's no wobble in the foot or knee. Many people need to focus on keeping weight on the inside part of the foot. Start with a small elevation of the non-standing leg. Progress to a 90-degree bend in the non-standing leg. Want to add an extra quad workout? Straighten the non-standing leg and bring it parallel to the ground with your hands overhead. This requires quad (thigh) strength in the non-standing leg.

Bent to Straight Leg Balance: This exercise tests the body's ability to control and stabilize a basic, dynamic movement in your lower chain. Start in a position that looks like the mid-stride of running. Keep your weight distributed through the sides, front, and back of your balancing foot. Then stand up straight with no wobble while keeping alignment. Return to the starting position and repeat five to 10 times.

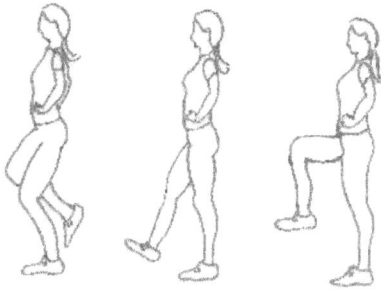

Forward Fold (touch toes): Try this move to gauge tightness in your lower back and hamstrings. Keep your weight equally distributed throughout the feet. Being far off here is a great indicator that you have been sitting for too long.

Good Mornings: This move tests lower and upper back muscles along with those in the back of the legs and is a good indicator of lower back, hip, and posture issues. You'll also see this exercise done with weights but don't start there. Stand with your feet hip distance apart. Ground through your feet. Bring your arms up so they are parallel to the ground, making a T with your torso. Fold forward while maintaining perfect upper body posture. Do not push this! Do it slowly. Take time to adjust. Try using something light like a broomstick or piece of PVC to help maintain upper body posture.

Clasped Hands Overhead Reaches: This exercise tests mobility limitations in the shoulders, neck, or upper back. Stand up straight. Raise your arms overhead. Clasp your hands together. Press and stretch up. Once straight, keep lifting up and push to the right, push up and to the left, then do a mini back bend in the middle. This is a great five to 10 second exercise. I do it multiple times a day to combat the effects of sitting. Take a picture from behind to see if your arms are straight.

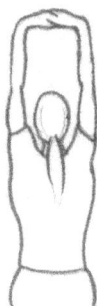

Clasped Hands Behind the Back Lifts: Try this move as a quick test to see if your chest and shoulders are tight. Or do it if you just want a quick stretch to combat seating. You can lift your arms away from your body if you have the mobility but don't force it. It's not necessary for many people to feel the benefits. When you advance in yoga, try this in combination with a forward fold. It's a basic exercise that I could not do for years. I told myself it was because I was a bigger guy. I can do it now, even if my range isn't as great compared to other people.

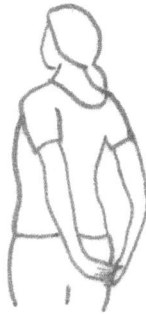

Lying Crossover Stretch (bent leg or straight leg): This move gauges your ability to rotate in the middle of your body (plus mobility in the back of the leg, if it's straight). This is one exercise that will make you feel better in a minute or two if you give it a chance. Lie on your back. Put your arms out to the side (making a T). Rotate your palms down and anchor your arms and palms to the floor. Lift your right leg.

- Option 1: Right leg is straight. This requires more hamstring mobility.

- Option 2: The right leg is bent at 90 degrees. Now rotate left and hold. For years, my right and left were imbalanced. If you are restricted here, it's a good time to have a conversation with a licensed professional to unlock that mobility. Take a picture and look for any major differences in your range of motion.

Malasana Pose: If the fitness industry ever comes up with a standard-ized structural health indicator test, I believe this pose will be on it.

If you can't do it, check for a lack of range of motion in your ankles, knees, hips, and/or back. In other words, it's a great and simple chain mobility test. This is a must-do pose in my life.

Slow Air Squats: This is a squat with no weight that tests the muscles you need to get up from a seated position. Three counts down. Three counts up. Take a picture from the side and compare to it to the proper form. A more advanced way to do this is with your arms overhead. It also tests mobility in your trunk and the strength and mobility of your upper back. Search for reliable information for "wall squats" as a modification or "basic glute max" or "quadriceps exercises" if this is challenging. If you have weak or unstable knees, try working on a bridge instead.

Bridge Pose: This pose is ideal for testing the strength of the glute max and lower back. I believe this pose, too, would make the list of red-flag indicators for basic strength. Lie on your back and move your feet as close to your butt as possible. Lift. You should not feel any pain. If you move your feet farther away from your butt and lift from your heels, it'll work the hamstrings more. Not being able to do this for at least five to 10 seconds with full range should be a sign that you need more strength training in the center (back) of your body.

Bird Dogs: This move tests shoulder-blade-connected muscles working together with pelvic-connected (core) muscles. This is a great indicator of core stability, including lower back (lumbar) strength and stability. Get on your hands and knees. Lift your straightened right leg and left arm. Do not rotate your hips. For a little extra test of strength and stability, tap the elbow of your lifted arm to the knee of your lifted leg. Then straighten them again. Go back and forth slowly with no wobble or pelvic rotation.[133]

Fire Hydrants: Use this exercise to test your ability to control and stabilize external rotation, hip extension, and outer hip muscles (abductors). Get on your hands and knees where your upper leg is perpendicular to the ground and your lower leg is parallel. Lift one leg at a time to the side. Hold it up, as high as possible, for one count. Lower and repeat. Be careful not to rotate your torso or hips too much.

Calf Raises (from three positions, with assistance from doorway or wall): These moves are great to gauge the strength of muscles that are critical for ankle function. Do these barefoot, and check for weight distribution through all toes, including the big toe. You can try it with your toes straight, toes inward, and toes outward. Take your time and try a small range of motion at a time. Use the wall, a chair, or the frame of a doorway for support.

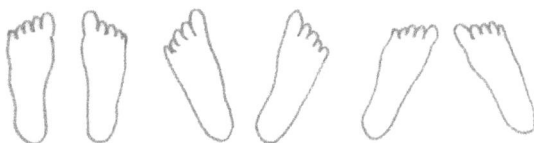

Wall Angels or Wall Snow Angels or Wall Slides (same exercise with many names): This move is great for testing the mobility of muscles that matter to posture. This is a great exercise to do for five to 30 seconds to combat the effect of sitting. If you aren't close here or you see lots of left-to-right imbalance, please seek assistance.

ADDITIONAL EXERCISES

Here are some other exercises to add to your list once you have the foundational moves down.

Slow Reverse Lunge to Balance: These lunges test lower body strength and its synergy with the upper body. Moving dynamically into a balanced position is an extended lower chain test. Please note that this is not to be done with sore or unstable knees, which require professional attention. I prefer the reverse lunge (versus the forward lunge) because it's easier to focus on form, and it's easier on the knees. Try it with your arms overhead to recruit more of the chain.

Doing this correctly, with full range and proper form, is not as simple as you may think. After the reverse lunge, bring the back leg forward to a 90-degree bend while standing upright. This tests your lower chain's ability to dynamically move into a balance.

Side Lunge to Side Leg Lift: I'm a huge fan of the side lunge. If you can do lots of exercises in the up-down plane of motion and can't do these, it's a sign that your program isn't diverse enough. This exercise dynamically recruits the outer and inner thighs and tests lower chain stability. Watch your posture, the alignment of your bent leg, and the anchoring of your foot on the non-bending leg. (It's always a good idea to find as many exercises as possible where you dynamically move in and out of balance, from as many directions as possible.)

Curtsy Lunge: This lunge helps gauge gluteus medius strength along with outer leg (TFL and IT band) tightness and general hip mobility. Do these slowly and do not force them. I would never do these quickly or with weights, and I would not suggest doing them often. Limitations or bad form can cause injury.

Note: If it's hard for you to reach a modest range of motion, as it was for me six years ago, there's something happening at the center of your body that needs correcting. I'm less concerned about your doing it perfectly with 100 percent range of motion. I'm more concerned if you can't get to 40 percent of the range. If you can do lots of heavy lifts like squats, dead lifts, or leg presses and you can't do this, it's a sign that your program isn't balanced, and it's time to have your weaknesses or limitations assessed and corrected.

Plank (on forearms or hands): Planks are great for checking the stability and strength of your key core. Add leg lifts for more of a challenge. Note: Whenever you perform plank exercises, watch out for elbow, shoulder, and neck/upper back issues and fix those issues first. Planks can be stressful on the neck if you have any problems or use bad form.

Side Plank (on forearm or hand): This type of plank gauges the stability and strength of the side core muscles. Add side leg lifts for more of a challenge.

Reverse Plank: This type of plank tests rear core muscles. For a more advanced option, see if you can lift up one leg at a time (keeping your hips as high as possible).

Please don't follow the cultural trend of spending most of your time working the front of your core, the muscles above the waist. The core is ALL the muscles that connect up and down from the pelvis.

BASIC YOGA POSES

I don't need to take yoga classes or dedicate an entire workout to yoga to integrate its value into my weekly routine. I figured out how to integrate the poses that are good for my body in small doses, regularly.

Child's Pose: Please learn this pose to relax and unwind. Do it with arms straight ahead, then reach right and left. With controlled breathing, it can be a great habit to relieve stress and prevent stress eating. It's a pose when you wake up in the morning or when you get home from work. And it's easy to do in a hotel room!

I may not have extreme flexibility today but the next two poses were impossible for me six months ago. I don't worry about doing them perfectly but I do them.

Easy Pose (Sukhasana): This pose helps to gauge basic hip and low back mobility. Get off the couch and hang out here with crossed legs while watching TV. If this is as uncomfortable for you as it was for me for a long time, hip mobility needs to be on your radar.

Kneeling (Thunderbolt Pose or Vajrasana): This pose focuses on ankle and knee mobility issues. If trying to slowly sit back on your feet hurts your ankles or knees, as it did for me, get checked by an expert. Don't push past any mild tightness in the knees or feet.

Low Lunge (Anjaneyasana): This pose tests hip flexor mobility. Press through the top of the back foot to work on ankle mobility.

Sun Salutations A and B: I can't tell you how doing these series of poses for just 30 seconds can make your body feel better. Doing these for a short time also can help you to stop thinking about yoga as only being a 60- or 90-minute activity. Learn the basics and take advantage of doing yoga in small doses. I'd rate Sun A and B among the most important exercises on this list. You can do several of these on each side in as little as three minutes, and it will help with mobility and breathing.

The basic poses of Sun Salutation A include:

- Upward Hand Pose: This is essentially lifting your hands overhead. I would modify this with a clasped-hands overhead press, as previously described.

- Forward Fold: See previous instruction.

- Chaturanga: Great for chest strength and triceps strength if you keep your elbows in. Get into plank position and lower slowly to the ground to test your upper body strength.

- Upward Dog: A great lower and upper back stretch. If you activate the top of your feet, you will work on foot mobility (plantar flexion).

- Down Dog: If done correctly, this opens the chest and shoulder muscles while testing the mobility in the back of your legs.

Chair Pose: This pose tests posture, ankle mobility, and thigh and butt strength. This is a great test to see if your scapular and shoulder-connected muscles are working equally on the left and right sides while you work your core muscles. If you are slouched forward and can't get your arms overhead, that's a great indicator that you lack strength and function in your upper back and shoulders. Try doing chair pose holding two cans (8.5 ounces each) or weights up to five pounds. Have someone take a picture of you from the rear and see if both arms look the same or if one is bent more than the other. I highly recommend that you work toward doing this on one leg at a time. This is a great way of working the full body.

Warrior I: One of the best exercises around, in my opinion. If you can do this with a full range of motion, hip rotation, and your feet anchored properly, that's a good indicator of head-to-toe strength. I prefer doing it with my hands clasped, pressing the arms straight up, to engage more posture-related muscles. At times, I sometimes do this pose for 30-60 seconds, holding light weights overhead as a warmup to my workout.

Make sure your rear foot is anchored, keeping pressure in the front, back and sides of feet. This is one of those exercises that completely changes when you focus on foot form. I see a lot of people have done yoga for years who don't get their front leg into a 90-degree bend or their torso rotated toward the front. If this is you, work with someone to get stronger glutes, quads (thighs), and more hip mobility. Figure out why you can't do this one if you can't. It is a great exercise.

Boat Pose: This pose is an indicator of core strength, using muscles above and below the pelvis. No slouching. Check upper body posture and alignment. Search for beginner's core exercises and upper back and scapular (shoulder blade) exercises if this move proves challenging.

Seated Pretzel (Lord of the Fishes Pose): This pose is great to highlight mobile hips working with a twisted spine, but it's very hard if you have trunk or hip mobility issues. This one took me a while. Keep the lower leg straight to modify this pose and ask a therapist or trainer for exercises to assist with getting here.

Revolved Crescent Lunge: This pose focuses on thigh and glute strength, hip flexor mobility, and trunk mobility. I'm a big fan. You may find this to be hard with hands in prayer position so keep your arms straight as a modification. The hand that is opposite your forward leg presses into the ground on the inside of the forward foot. Twist your torso and lift the opposite arm to the sky.

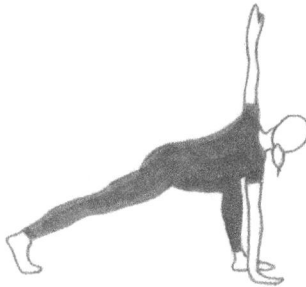

Triangle Pose: This pose will stretch your feet, knees, hips, groin, spine, shoulders, and chest while working on strengthening your core as long as you use the proper form. Get into this pose slowly.

Revolved Triangle Pose: This is an advanced pose. It should probably be on the advanced list, but I simply believe in it. This is one where 100 percent may be far away. Advancing from 20 percent of full range can be a great goal. It's an unbelievable indicator of health because it stabilizes the feet through a twisted core. It took me years to get here. Search for IT band and TFL stretches along with trunk and hip mobility exercises to work your way up to this. I didn't get proficient by doing yoga in classes, where an instructor may have you in this position for up to 20 or 30 seconds in a 60- or 90-minute class, if it's done at all. I used this as a warmup exercise for all of my workouts for months. This is an example of learning yoga in class and expanding it to other parts of your life.

Warrior III Pose: This is a full body test, requiring ankle and lower chain stability, core strength, and control of scapular-connected muscles. This one is hard, too, but I believe in balancing exercises. Modify with T arms or hands in prayer position versus the (harder) superman arm option. Look for as little hip rotation as possible. Perfect form may take years, or you may never get there. But it's always worth trying. Work on single leg dead lifts without weight to build up to this.

Single Leg Dead Lift (from balancing while standing upright): Do you know how to do yoga Warrior III or a modification with hands at prayer position or T arms? Can you balance on one leg while the non-weight-bearing leg is straight out in front of you (parallel to the ground)? Now move back and forth from one position to the other.

PILATES BASICS

I believe Pilates "swimmers" and prone snow angels may be among the best and most underappreciated exercises to test the back of the core and the muscles that connect to the shoulder blade. When many people "work the core," they are on their back. Exercising in different positions, though, is how health happens.

Swimmers: If you take this from a "can't do" to "can do" for 20 seconds or more, the back of your body will thank you. Keep the legs close together. There are alternatives to swimmers to work more posture and shoulder blade-connected muscles from your belly, or prone position. You can try swimmers with thumbs facing up versus palms down. Without moving the legs, you can make your arms like a Y and move them up and down with thumbs up. You also can place your arms in a T and lift them up with palms down. There are lots of great exercises to do from your belly to work the rear chain from the neck to the knees. They are among the most ignored in fitness programs. Core workouts aren't just on the back. Make sure you work from prone position and on the sides.

Prone Snow Angels: Did you ever do a snow angel on your back when you were a kid? Well, for this one, get on your belly, and do it with your arms and legs lifted as high as possible. Start in a swimmer pose: Your legs are together and arms are straight out in front of you with palms down. Lift your arms and legs and keep them lifted as high as possible. Now move your legs out, making a Y with your legs. Sweep your arms out, moving them to the side of your body with palms up. The challenge is to keep lifting your hands and feet as high as possible while moving them from over your head to your side.

Scissors: This is a dynamic core exercise that will also test hamstring mobility.

Lying Crossovers: This is like the previous lying cross over stretch, but it's dynamic and involves trunk rotation plus core mobility.

*Pilates Side Serie*s: These exercises highlight strength and control of the side core muscles as you move the legs with varying leg rotation—straight, internal, and external. Lie on the ground on one side, then do leg lifts with neutral (straight) foot (flexed), leg circles, up-and-over taps with heel down (external leg rotation), up-and-over taps with toe down (internal leg rotation), and lower leg lifts (to test inner thigh). Find a way to learn these from a pro. If you exercise a lot and can't do eight to 10 reps without rest, consider diversifying your routine.

Pilates Saw: When you do this with proper spine alignment and rotation, this exercise with a twist tests the back of your body. This is more than sitting down with your legs wide and touching your toes and may require some coaching. Do not slouch your upper back to reach farther. Keep your spine upright as you fold forward and twist.

Side Clams (on your side, from forearm): Have you mastered fire hydrants? Now engage the core muscles on the side of the body.

These exercises may seem like a lot, so divide and conquer them, a few at a time. Some are harder than others and some involve only stretching. If you focused on just three exercises in a 60-day window, starting with the easier ones first, you can make enormous progress in two years. If you focused on six exercises in a 60-day window, you'll see great progress in just one year. If you hired a personal coach, you'll see results even more quickly.

I hope that you research the list above for no other reason than to learn how to put a program together that uses all parts of the body in all directions. Use this list with exercises you learn from others, like therapists and trainers, to build your list of exercises that will test your body from head to toe with low force using your natural body weight.

Harder exercises to test your body or your kids who prefer sports or high force exercises:

If you're looking for a further challenge to test your head-to-toe chain before doing higher force exercises like running, heavy lifting, or playing sports, try these and exercises like them.

Pilates options for those who do high force exercises or sports:

Pilates Teasers: Got yoga boat pose down? Now move in and out dynamically.

Pilates Side Series (from side plank on elbow): When you master the side plank and the Pilates side series, you can move on to combine them. Leg lifts, leg circles, and up-and-over taps are much harder when done from the side plank position. Want to add the upper body and shoulder stability? Do them while supporting with a straight arm instead of your elbow.

Single Leg Bridge Pose (with leg lifts): This is bridge pose with one foot on the ground and the other lifted vertically. Move the non-weight-bearing leg up and down.

Yoga options for those who do high force exercises or sports:

Single Leg Figure Four Chair Pose: Combine figure four with a chair pose. This will test your ability to balance in dorsiflexion (moving the foot up toward the shin) while working on hip mobility and key core muscles. Reach your arms up and back to make this a full body exercise.

Single Leg Down Dog to Plank Knee Taps: These are common moves in yoga classes. Work on them outside of class to get the most out of your practice. Try to get to a point where you can tap your knee to one elbow. Do a single leg down dog, then tap the opposite elbow. Tapping the elbow, or higher up on the triceps, is a great test of core strength.

If you want more of an upper body challenge, do a spider push up when tapping your right leg to your right elbow (or left to left).

Half-Moon Pose: To do this without a block requires lots and lots of stability from the foot through the entire core, enlisting more of the side muscles than in Warrior III.

Fallen Triangle Pose (with lower leg lift): If you want a challenging core exercise that adds an inner thigh test, this one is for you. Master the pose without the leg lift before adding this one. This is also a great upper body strength and shoulder stability test.

If you skipped *Revolved Triangle* in the first list, add it here.

Functional exercises for those who do exercises or sports:

Twisting Balance: Balance on one leg with the non-standing leg bent at 90 degrees. Extend both arms straight in front of you holding something like a yoga block or book (about eight to 12 inches in size). Twist left until torso faces 90 degrees from center. Twist right. Repeat. This will test a pattern of muscles from the bottom of your feet through and across the core. Advance to holding a light weight.

Side (lateral) Lunge to Wood Chop: A classic. Do a side lunge holding a weight or ball, starting with something really light, then dynamically move the weight or ball while rotating the body.

Work with a good trainer to find as many dynamic and explosive twisting exercises as possible.

Alternating Arm and Leg Lifts (from plank position): Don't abandon Pilates swimmers because this is different. Getting in a plank and lifting each arm with the opposite leg, pausing for a while, and repeating is a great functional test for athletes.

Calf Raises from Three Angles (see previous instructions) without assistance from the wall: Full range with pause at the top. Add hands clasped and lifted overhead for more challenge. Focus on weight distributed through all toes.

Twisted Rear Lunge to Frankenstein Kicks: Lunge backward, and twist over the forward leg. Then dynamically move into a Frankenstein kick.

Work with a trainer to find more explosive functional exercises like this if you play sports.

Single Leg Squats (or pistons): Want to lift a lot of weight? Why not test your ability to lift your body weight on one leg first. You'll know if you have any imbalances and lower chain instability.

Single Leg Squat to Warrior I: This is a great strength-training combo exercise.

Windmill: Have you mastered yoga's triangle pose? You can find this exercise by searching for "kettlebell windmill" but you don't need a kettlebell. DO NOT start with weight until you master the basic move.

Now make it dynamic and add some weight. Move up and down, first by keeping your lower arm sliding along your leg. Try to get to a point where you don't have to touch your leg as your torso goes from perpendicular to parallel (relative to the ground). Add weight when you progress. Start with a small amount: Less than two pounds. An 8.5 oz can of food is a good place to start.

Slow Side Kick: Master yoga's half-moon pose? Work on a side kick. Face forward. Do a side kick to the back of the room, then pause at the end. Take at least five seconds from start to finish. This is a great test of lower chain stability, core strength, and core mobility.

These exercises are some of the ways I check my body and maintain good, holistic health. But there are many more exercises at lower levels, at higher levels, and everywhere in between.

Find them.

Build your list at your level.

Keep evolving it.

Your whole body will thank you.

Endnotes

1   https://www.boneandjointburden.org/docs/BMUS%20Impact%20of%20MSK%20
    on%20Americans%20booklet_4th%20Edition%20%282018%29.pdf

2   https://www.forbes.com/sites/niallmccarthy/2015/06/25/the-biggest-military-budgets-
    as-a-percentage-of-gdp-infographic-2/#1f4d9c364c47

3   https://www.health.harvard.edu/blog/surgeon-generals-1964-report-making-smoking-
    history-201401106970

4   https://www.bicycling.com/training/a20025230/three-stretches-for-tight-hips/

5   https://www.bicycling.com/training/g20035207/7-ways-you-re-hurting-your-knees/

6   https://sportfactoryproshop.com/blog/how-to-get-rid-of-cycling-neck-and-shoulder-
    pain-/

7   https://health.gov/paguidelines/second-edition/

8   https://www.cdc.gov/nchs/fastats/obesity-overweight.htm

9   https://www.boneandjointburden.org/docs/BMUS%20Impact%20of%20MSK%20
    on%20Americans%20booklet_4th%20Edition%20%282018%29.pdf

10 https://www.builtlean.com/2012/09/24/body-fat-percentage-men-women/

11 https://www.acefitness.org/education-and-resources/lifestyle/tools-calculators/percent-
    body-fat-calculator

12 https://www.allmaxnutrition.com/post-articles/supplements/diuretics-in-
    bodybuilding-the-good-the-bad-the-tragic/

13 https://www.lifehacker.com.au/2015/09/how-fitness-models-really-get-those-
    photoshoot-bodies/

14 https://greatist.com/connect/truth-behind-fitness-photo-shoots#7

15 https://tntnutrition.org/eating-after-fitness-competitions-healing-your-relationship-
    with-food/

16 https://1stphorm.com/blog/the-detrimental-effects-of-post-contest-bingeing-and-how-
    to-fight-back/

17   Sara J. Solnick and David Hemenway, "Is more always better?: A survey on positional concerns," *Journal of Economic Behavior & Organization*, Vol. 37 (1998): 373-383.

18   https://www.albany.edu/~gs149266/Solnick%20&%20Hemenway%20(1998)%20-%20Positional%20concerns.pdf

19   Victoria Medvec, Thomas Gilovich and Scott Madey, "When Less Is More: Counterfactual Thinking and Satisfaction Among Olympic Medalists," *Journal of Personality and Social Psychology*, Vol. 69, No. 4, (1995): 603-61.

20   https://www.commonsensemedia.org/children-teens-body-image-media-infographic

21   https://www.ncbi.nlm.nih.gov/pmc/articles/PMC2530935/

22   https://www.nationaleatingdisorders.org/learn/by-eating-disorder/other/orthorexia

23   https://www.eatingdisorderhope.com/information/orthorexia-excessive-exercise/exercise-bulimia-and-drunkorexia-the-lesser-known-disorders

24   https://www.mayoclinic.org/diseases-conditions/bulimia/symptoms-causes/syc-20353615

25   https://results.nyrr.org/event/700913/overview

26   https://runningmagazine.ca/sections/runs-races/celebrities-running-the-2019-tcs-new-york-city-marathon/

27   https://www.cdc.gov/nchs/products/databriefs/db288.htm

28   https://www.cdc.gov/nchs/fastats/obesity-overweight.htm

29   https://nypost.com/2018/06/28/exercise-and-obesity-are-somehow-both-rising/

30   http://www.med.unc.edu/www/newsarchive/2009/february/chronic-low-back-pain-on-the-rise-unc-study-finds-alarming-increase-in-prevalence

31   https://www.ninds.nih.gov/Disorders/Patient-Caregiver-Education/Fact-Sheets/Low-Back-Pain-Fact-Sheet

32   https://www.washingtonpost.com/news/morning-mix/wp/2014/11/20/text-neck-is-becoming-an-epidemic-and-could-wreck-your-spine/

33   https://www.goodhousekeeping.com/health/wellness/a26555846/text-neck-back-pain-kids/

34   https://thesocietypages.org/socimages/2012/02/27/torches-of-freedom-women-and-smoking-propaganda/

35   https://www.cbsnews.com/pictures/outrageous-vintage-cigarette-ads/6/

36   https://thesocietypages.org/socimages/2009/08/24/marketing-cigarettes-to-me/

37   https://www.healthcare-administration-degree.net/10-evil-vintage-cigarette-ads-promising-better-health/

38   https://www.health.harvard.edu/blog/surgeon-generals-1964-report-making-smoking-history-201401106970

39   https://www.ncbi.nlm.nih.gov/pmc/articles/PMC3894634/

40   https://www.ncbi.nlm.nih.gov/pmc/articles/PMC1759327/pdf/v003p00130.pdf

41   https://www.cdc.gov/tobacco/data_statistics/by_topic/policy/legislation/index.htm

42   https://www.heart.org/en/news/2019/01/31/cardiovascular-diseases-affect-nearly-half-of-american-adults-statistics-show

43   https://www.acefitness.org/education-and-resources/lifestyle/tools-calculators/heart-rate-zone-calculator

44   https://www.heart.org/en/healthy-living/fitness/fitness-basics/target-heart-rates

45   https://www.cedars-sinai.org/blog/texting-thumb.html

46   http://www.thespinehealthinstitute.com/news-room/health-blog/how-high-heels-affect-your-body

47   https://barefootstrongblog.com/2014/12/02/big-toe-biomechanics/

48   https://sbrsport.me/2013/03/31/big-toe-big-job/

49   https://www.issaonline.com/blog/index.cfm/2018/how-does-sitting-impact-my-posture

50   https://www.spineuniverse.com/wellness/ergonomics/sitting-disease-its-impact-your-spine

51   https://www.washingtonpost.com/news/morning-mix/wp/2014/11/20/text-neck-is-becoming-an-epidemic-and-could-wreck-your-spine/

52   https://www.healthline.com/health/fitness-exercise/text-neck-treatment

53   Evan Osar, *The Psoas Solution: The Practitioner's Guide to Rehabilitation, Corrective Exercise, and Training for Improved Function* (North Atlantic Books 2017).

54   https://www.drnorthrup.com/psoas-muscle-vital-muscle-body/

55   https://www.stack.com/a/psoas-muscle

56   https://www.menshealth.com/health/a19532915/biggest-running-myth-debunked/

57   https://www.nbcsports.com/chicago/bulls/derrick-rose-if-load-management-would-have-been-around-i-probably-would-have-still-been

58   https://www.kcur.org/post/not-sync-his-body-lorenzo-cain-finds-new-way-run#stream/0

59   Dr. Andreo Spina. "How incorrect pull up technique can lead to medial elbow pain." https://www.youtube.com/watch?v=tiW2BuxKT84

60   https://www.huffpost.com/entry/sexy-equinox-ad-bethesda_n_3535059

61   I. A. Kapandji MD, *The Physiology of the Joints, Volume 3* (Churchill Livingstone, 2008)

62   https://www.ucsfhealth.org/conditions/ankle_sprain/

63   https://www.ncbi.nlm.nih.gov/pubmedhealth/PMH0072735/

64   https://www.runnersworld.com/health-injuries/a20803577/get-healthy-calves-and-shins/

65   https://www.mountainpeakfitness.com/blog/strength-stability-foot-ankle-lower-leg

66   https://www.verywellhealth.com/ankle-exercises-a-complete-guide-2696480

67   https://www.orthocarolina.com/media/improving-balance-for-all-ages-focusing-on-ankle-stability

68   https://running.pocketoutdoormedia.com/3-ways-to-increase-running-cadence-for-speed_112765

69   https://www.webmd.com/healthy-aging/guide/sarcopenia-with-aging#1

70   https://www.health.harvard.edu/staying-healthy/preserve-your-muscle-mass

71   https://health.gov/paguidelines/second-edition/pdf/Physical_Activity_Guidelines_2nd_edition.pdf

72   https://www.acefitness.org/about-ace/press-room/press-releases/7141/ace-applauds-revisions-to-the-physical-activity-guidelines-for-americans

73   https://www.ncbi.nlm.nih.gov/pubmed/22777332

74   https://www.webmd.com/fitness-exercise/features/get-more-burn-from-your-workout#1

75   https://www.nbcchicago.com/news/local/History-of-the-Bank-of-America-Shamrock-Shuffle-8K-370010941.html

76   https://www.aarp.org/health/conditions-treatments/info-2018/tommy-john-opposes-namesake-surgery.html

77   https://www.ncbi.nlm.nih.gov/pmc/articles/PMC4805849/

78   https://www.ace-pt.org/core-strength-young-athletes/

79   https://well.blogs.nytimes.com/2015/12/30/can-too-much-exercise-harm-the-heart/

80   https://globalnews.ca/news/3810972/too-much-high-intensity-exercise-can-be-bad-for-your-heart-study-says/

81   https://www.elsevier.com/about/press-releases/research-and-journals/high-levels-of-intense-exercise-may-be-unhealthy-for-the-heart2

82   https://www.bbc.com/news/health-50181155

83   https://www.doyouyoga.com/5-famous-athletes-who-do-yoga-49478/

84   https://www.masslive.com/redsox/2017/02/david_price_chris_sale_other_r.html

85   https://www.baltimoresun.com/maryland/carroll/news/ph-cc-youth-sports-health-hw-20160403-story.html

86   https://wwws.fitnessrepublic.com/fitness/when-to-push-through-pain-injury.html

87   https://www.hopkinsmedicine.org/orthopaedic-surgery/about-us/ask-the-experts/pain.html

88   https://www.cnn.com/2017/11/27/health/marathon-training-injury-exercise-jampolis/index.html

89   https://www.nytimes.com/2018/08/22/well/move/how-you-felt-about-gym-class-may-impact-your-exercise-habits-today.html

90   https://www.theatlantic.com/education/archive/2019/01/why-pe-is-terrible/581467/

91   https://www.emarketer.com/content/emarketer-total-media-ad-spending-worldwide-will-rise-7-4-in-2018

92   https://thebrain.mcgill.ca/flash/i/i_07/i_07_p/i_07_p_tra/i_07_p_tra.html

93 L. Boroditsky, L. Schmidt and W. Phillips, *Sex, Syntax, and Semantics*. *In Language in mind: Advances in the study of language and cognition*, Gentner & S. Goldin-Meadow, pp. 61- 80. Cambridge University Press.

94 https://contently.com/2016/04/14/dangerous-power-emotional-advertising/

95 https://www.psychologytoday.com/us/blog/inside-the-consumer-mind/201302/how-emotions-influence-what-we-buy

96 https://www.nielsen.com/us/en/

97 https://www.cnbc.com/2018/11/08/cdc-says-smoking-rates-fall-to-record-low-in-us.html

98 https://www.scientificamerican.com/article/why-does-the-brain-need-s/

99 http://news.mit.edu/2005/habit

100 https://charlesduhigg.com/how-companies-learn-your-secrets-part-1/

101 https://charlesduhigg.com

102 https://jamesclear.com

103 https://gretchenrubin.com/books/

104 https://www.forbes.com/sites/forbescoachescouncil/2018/06/22/15-proven-strategies-for-building-and-dropping-habits/#139dc82f5872

105 https://www.developgoodhabits.com/how-to-form-a-habit-in-8-easy-steps/

106 https://jamesclear.com/habit-triggers

107 https://charlesduhigg.com/how-habits-work/

108 https://www.healthline.com/nutrition/how-food-addiction-works

109 https://www.ncbi.nlm.nih.gov/pmc/articles/PMC4769029/

110 https://www.forbes.com/sites/alicegwalton/2011/06/16/penetrating-postures-the-science-of-yoga/#64a5f7297d4b

111 https://www.ncbi.nlm.nih.gov/pubmed/29278839

112 https://www.psychologytoday.com/us/blog/your-neurochemical-self/201608/stop-anxiety-adjusting-expectations

113 https://www.medicalnewstoday.com/articles/319157.php

114 https://www.webmd.com/depression/guide/exercise-depression#1

115 https://simonsinek.com/about/?ref=footer

116 https://jamesclear.com/identity-based-habits

117 https://news.gallup.com/poll/224336/eight-americans-afflicted-stress.aspx

118 https://www.sleephealth.org/sleep-health/the-state-of-sleephealth-in-america/

119 https://adaa.org/about-adaa/press-room/facts-statistics

120 https://www.aafp.org/news/health-of-the-public/20180219nchsdepression.html

121 https://policyoptions.irpp.org/2015/05/25/exercise-is-the-worlds-best-drug-but-its-not-a-weight-loss-drug/

122   http://news.mit.edu/2005/habit

123   https://www.acefitness.org/education-and-resources/lifestyle/blog/5073/8-reasons-hiit-
      workouts-are-so-effective

124   https://health.ucdavis.edu/sportsmedicine/resources/vo2description.html

125   https://www.webmd.com/depression/ss/slideshow-avoid-foods-anxiety-depression

126   https://www.huffingtonpost.com.au/2017/07/16/the-best-and-worst-foods-to-eat-
      when-youre-stressed_a_23029130/

127   https://www.health.harvard.edu/mind-and-mood/relaxation-techniques-breath-
      control-helps-quell-errant-stress-response

128   https://science.howstuffworks.com/life/sleep-obesity1.htm

129   https://www.sleep.org/articles/eat-to-sleep-better/

130   https://www.health.harvard.edu/mind-and-mood/relaxation-techniques-breath-
      control-helps-quell-errant-stress-response

131   https://www.sciencedaily.com/releases/2018/05/180510101254.htm

132   https://www.forbes.com/sites/daviddisalvo/2017/11/29/how-breathing-calms-your-
      brain-and-other-science-based-benefits-of-controlled-breathing/#3dcb9a082221

133   https://www.acefitness.org/education-and-resources/lifestyle/exercise-library/14/bird-
      dog

www.ingramcontent.com/pod-product-compliance
Lightning Source LLC
Chambersburg PA
CBHW020252030426
42336CB00010B/728